The Impotence Sourcebook

by
Christopher P. Steidle, M.D.

Foreword by
John J. Mulcahy, M.D., Ph.D., F.A.C.S.

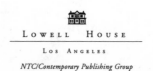

LOWELL HOUSE

LOS ANGELES

NTC/Contemporary Publishing Group

The treatments presented herein are in no way intended to diagnose or treat medical or physical problems or to be used as a substitute for medical treatment or counseling.

Library of Congress Cataloging-in-Publication Data

Steidle, Christopher P.
    The impotence sourcebook / by Christopher P. Steidle.
       p. cm.
    Includes index.
    ISBN 0-7373-0252-6 (paper)
    1. Impotence—Popular works.   I. Title.
  RC889.S686   1998
  616.6'92—dc21   98-5062
                                 CIP

Published by Lowell House
A division of NTC/Contemporary Publishing Group, Inc.
4255 West Touhy Avenue
Lincolnwood (Chicago), Illinois 60646-1975 U.S.A.

Printed and bound in the United States of America

International Standard Book Number: 0-7373-0252-6

99 00 01 02 03 04 DHD 18 17 16 15 14 13 12 11 10 9 8 7 6 5 4 3 2 1

This book is dedicated to my family: My wife, Jean, and my sons, John and Stephen, who have been of the utmost support through this endeavor. My father and mother, Walter and Dorothy. Finally, to my patients, many of whom have become my friends and my inspiration for continuing to work.

ACKNOWLEDGMENTS

I am very grateful to Dr. John Mulcahy for providing his review of the manuscript and writing the foreword. It was his enthusiasm and expertise in this field that fueled my interest. I would never have undertaken or completed this project without his guidance over the last fifteen years. Special thanks to Dr. Raymond C. Rosen for the use of the erectile dysfunction questionnaire and interpretation.

I wish to thank Chip and Ralphie Blasius for their tremendous assistance in helping me to complete this manuscript.

I also wish to thank my editor, Bud Sperry, and managing editor, Maria Magallanes, for being so patient with a first-time author.

CONTENTS

Foreword

Erectile dysfunction is a common problem associated with both the aging process and diseases and injuries that affect the blood flow into the penis. It is estimated that one in four men in their late fifties suffer from this condition; almost half of men in their sixties are impotent; and most men in their seventies are impotent. As longevity increases, more couples will advance to the age when they may be affected by erectile dysfuntion. The baby boom generation is now progressing into their sixth decade, where unreliable erections begin to take an emotional toll. Progressive attitudes regarding sexuality among this population indicate that there will be a great demand for treatment as we approach the new millennium.

Today, a variety of treatments for erectile dysfunction are available so that virtually anyone who is motivated to continue with sexual activity would be considered a candidate for successful treatment. Such was not the case thirty years ago when most erectile dysfunction was thought to be psychogenic or situational in nature and attitudes toward sex were more puritanical. Discussion of sex was frowned upon, and its presentation by the media was minimal and certainly not graphic. Anyone who applied for a research grant in the area of sexual dysfunction was simply regarded as a pervert. Likewise, the treatment for impotence was limited to a cold shower to alleviate sexual frustration.

The first effective therapy introduced in the early 1970s was the penile implant. As the effectiveness of implants became evident, patients began to come forward for therapy, and a true appreciation of the magnitude of the problem evolved. This provided the impetus for the development of a variety of treatments. Changing attitudes toward sexuality, more open discussion of sexual problems, and presentation in the media occurred simultaneously and certainly aided this development. Now, in addition to penile implants we have vacuum devices and various medications to supplement waning erections. Dr. Chris Steidle has participated in the development of many of these advance treatments, and this book certainly reflects his experience and practical approach to the problem.

The Impotence Sourcebook is well-organized and starts with the normal process of the erection and what occurs in its development. This is followed by a discussion of the tests available with an emphasis on selective work-up. Because this field is rife with abuse of services, the warnings that Dr. Steidle gives throughout the book are pertinent. Not all patients need to undergo every test for an appropriate treatment of their particular problem. Heeding his advice will, in many cases, avoid much unnecessary testing and treatments which may be ineffective.

The book cites several clinical examples culled from the author's own experience which help solidify its concepts. As Dr. Steidle progresses to the various treatments, he provides preventive tips on sexual health. In addition to erectile dysfunction, sections on ejaculatory dysfunction and penile enlargement are enlightening as research in these areas are undergoing investigation, and new treatments for problems are now becoming available. Many men are fixated on the size of the penis; some become emotionally involved over what they believe are aberrations. At the end of each chapter, a unique summary highlights the important points.

The area of sexual dysfunction is ready to mushroom into a commonly treated problem as less aggressive treatments such as oral medications become available. Particularly helpful for the reader is the warning about clinics who advertise widely, test extensively, charge exorbitantly, and offer limited treatment options. This book provides practical advice on the diagnosis and treatment of erectile dysfunction and its associated disorders.

—JOHN J. MULCAHY, M.D., PH.D., F.A.C.S.

INTRODUCTION

One of the most devastating things that can happen to a man is the unexpected loss of an erection during sexual intercourse. Erectile dysfunction is frightening and embarrassing, and because men have been taught early on not to talk about their genitals and sexual functioning, they frequently do not know where to turn for help. In fact, most men's sexual knowledge is acquired secondhand from adolescent peers. This knowledge is also supported by such "textbooks" as adult magazines and pornographic videos, which are woefully inaccurate and misleading and tend to give most men the impression that intercourse is a superhuman event enjoyed by people with abnormally sized genitals.

Impotence is defined as the inability to achieve and maintain an erection to permit satisfactory sexual intercourse. Because of the negative connotations of the term *impotence*, we have now substituted the term *erectile dysfunction*. Erectile dysfunction is a more accurate term because, typically, men who have erectile dysfunction may still be able to perform sexually by foreplay and oral sex, although not necessarily by vaginal penetration. Men with erectile dysfunction may also retain the ability to ejaculate, even with a flaccid penis.

Erectile dysfunction is deceptively common. It has been estimated that 66 percent of men by the age of seventy are affected by erectile dysfunction. In other words, only a third of men by the age of seventy are still able to achieve an erection sufficient enough for vaginal penetration. The largest study of its type ever conducted, the Massachusetts Male Aging Study examined and questioned a large group of men between the ages of forty and seventy about sexuality, and some interesting facts appeared. Although well-known among most health-care professionals, many men would find it surprising that cigarette smoking is a major risk factor for the loss of erections. Among men with heart disease who smoke cigarettes, 56 percent were impotent, compared with 21 percent of nonsmokers. If this statistic were printed on the side of cigarette packages, men would probably think harder about smoking.

In the study, the prevalence of impotence of all degrees was estimated at 52 percent. Based on the U.S. population, this would be equivalent to 18 million American men. Men with diabetes were three times more likely to have erectile dysfunction than those without diabetes, regardless of whether they were insulin dependent or non-insulin dependent. Heart disease, high blood pressure, and a low level of high-density lipoproteins (HDL, the "good" form of cholesterol) correlated strongly with impotence as well. The higher the HDL, the lower the risk of erectile dysfunction. For older men with HDL levels greater than 90, no erectile dysfunction was identified. Perhaps if this statistic were printed on food labels, it might encourage people to adopt low-fat diets.

Another interesting finding was that certain psychological factors were strongly associated with erectile dysfunction including depression and anger, repressed or outwardly expressed. Anger and hostility are associated with certain other medical conditions, such as ulcers and coronary artery disease, but this is the first time it has been found to be related to erectile dysfunction as well.

As a board-certified urologist in active clinical practice,

I am amazed by the phenomenal changes in the treatment of erectile dysfunction that have occurred during the last decade and even in the last two years. While completing my training, physicians had very little to offer patients other than penile implants and ineffectual oral medications. Little scientific knowledge was available about how erections happen, and most erectile dysfunction was diagnosed as psychological. A typical medical workup consisted of telling men to wrap postage stamps around their penis, and if they woke up and the stamps were broken, this indicated that the condition was psychological and was treated accordingly. To this day, many patients still say to me, "I'm not sure if this is in my head, but . . ."

Over the last decade, however, the field of urology has undergone a renaissance. We now know that the vast majority of men with erectile dysfunction have organic disease and, in fact, a minimal psychological component. From a clinical standpoint, I can frequently identify several risk factors by taking a careful history and physical and make a strong, positive impact on the man's life. I find it very gratifying to treat men with erectile dysfunction and am always amazed at the instant improvement in self-confidence when sexual functioning is restored.

By the year 2000 a series of oral medications will be available to treat erectile dysfunction. We not only will be able to treat male erectile dysfunction, but also female sexual dysfunction. The study of female sexual dysfunction is also undergoing a phenomenal renaissance. Many old myths are being completely transformed and information that physicians once treated as sacred has been proven to be completely without scientific merit. We will eventually discover the exact causes of erectile dysfunction. This will make a tremendous difference in the quality of people's lives.

About This Book

The purpose of this book will be how to recognize the problem (if it exists), how to prevent the problem, and how to maintain good erections for life.

This book will explore many preventable risk factors and some lifestyles that promote good sexual health. I will also discuss what you should expect from a health-care professional in terms of a medical history and physical examination, as well as what treatment options are currently available. We will also address some of the more unusual problems seen in the management of men with sexual dysfunction and, finally, new developments in this field. Many of the products soon to be released in the near future will forever change how men with erectile dysfunction are managed.

I will summarize each chapter in a series of take-home points. These are the thoughts that are the most important and the most beneficial. Additionally, each chapter highlights case studies from my professional experience to illustrate both the problem and the solution.

Chapter 1

Anatomy and Physiology

Anatomy

The penis is made up of three separate cylinders (see Figure 1.1). The two paired cylinders called the *corpora cavernosa* make up the majority of the bulk and the erectile functioning of the penis. Both these cylinders actually communicate with each other for approximately three-quarters of their length through small holes between the cylinders. (This is why penile injections are applied into only one shaft or cylinder of the penis.) As the penis approaches the body, these two cylinders split and are anchored to the pelvic bone by a tough membrane. Each of these cylinders is encased in a very tough thick sheath called the *tunica albuginea*. A tough thick membrane surrounds the penis so that when it is filled with

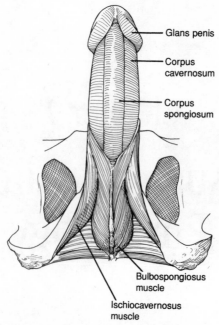

Figure 1.1. Frontal view of the penis.
Vivus, Inc.

blood under pressure it creates a firm structure that allows penetration.

The third cylinder of the penis is called the *corpus spongiosum*, and it contains the urethra. The tissue around this erectile body is much thinner, and the cylinder actually sits in a groove created by the other two cylinders. As this structure approaches the end of the penis, it becomes swollen and is known as the *glans*, or the head of the penis. As this layer gets closer to the body, it expands to form the *bulb*. Covering all three of these cylinders is a thick tough membrane called *Buck's fascia*. Finally, a final layer covers this area called *Colles fascia*, or the superficial layer. This is actually continuous with the abdominal wall and makes this whole supporting struc-

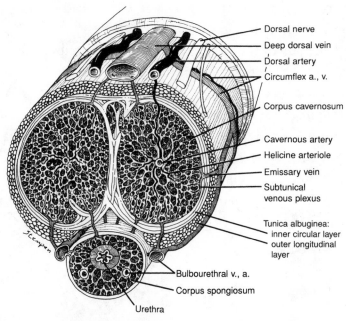

Figure 1.2. Cross-section of the penis.
Vivus, Inc.

ture of the penis very tough, allowing it to take quite a bit of force and trauma.

The skin covering the penis is extremely mobile and expandable. This is necessary to allow an erection to take place. The skin of the penis is unique in this property, and it is controlled by the hormonal system. The head of the penis, or the glans, is an anatomically distinct structure covered by a foreskin. This is a double layer of penile skin that is very freely moveable. Because of its movability and expandability, it is very sensitive to any degree of swelling or trauma. It is for this reason that the skin of the penis can become massively swollen even with minimal trauma in a short period of time. For instance, a bee sting or spider bite to the penis can produce massive swelling and actually distort the penis to the point where the head of the penis is no longer visible.

The body of the penis is anchored to the pubic bone, and a thickening of the rectus muscle anchors the top of the penis. The rectus muscles, or "abs," are the muscles in the middle of the abdominal wall. This thickened layer, called the fundiform ligament, extends off the rectus muscle to anchor the penis. When this ligament is cut, as in so-called penis-lengthening operations, the penis may appear longer although it simply hangs lower from the body because it is disattached.

Blood Supply

The blood supply of the penis comes from a main blood vessel that goes down the back of the body called the aorta. The aorta then branches to an internal and external iliac artery, and finally a pudendal artery passes underneath the pelvic bone and terminates in the common penile artery. When sitting and especially when riding a bicycle, a man can cut off blood circulation to this common penile artery. When this artery is damaged, arterial insufficiency and subsequent erectile dysfunction occur. A cavernosal artery supplies blood into each of the erectile bodies of the penis.

The blood supply to the glans, or head, of the penis is part of a separate system. It is for this reason that men can achieve an erection without swollen glans, such as in conditions known as *priapism* (see chapter 5). This is also true for men who have penile implants; the glans or head of the penis will not become enlarged.

The underlying mechanism of an erection is the corporo-veno-occlusive mechanism. When the veins cannot become compressed or blocked, an erection cannot be maintained. Without this very sensitive mechanism, blood leaks prematurely from the penis and produces the loss of an erection. This type of erectile dysfunction is called a *venous leak*.

Nervous System

The nervous system of the penis is involved with both the creation and maintenance of an erection as well as an ejaculation. The most numerous sensory nerves are located on the head, or glans, of the penis. To achieve an erection it takes multiple input from numerous areas of both the brain and the spinal cord. The first part of a penile erection is controlled by the brain, known as a *psychogenic erection*. This occurs under any type of mental or erotic stimulation. Penile erections can also be caused by friction of the skin of the penis alone. This is known as a *reflexogenic erection,* which commonly occurs among men who have had damage to the spinal cord and who are unable to get an erection unless physically stimulated.

Sperm

The scrotum is a unique structure with very thin, loose skin that is slightly hair bearing. It is also controlled by the endocrine system and functions as a receptacle for the testes. Keeping the testicles outside the body produces a cooler environment and thus provides the best area for *spermatogenesis*, or the creation of sperm, to take place. Warmth tends to prevent sperm from developing properly. Underlying the skin of the scrotum is the *cremasteric muscle*. This muscle is incorporated into the scrotum and by contracting, it elevates the testicles. This is done in response to cool and warm weather and noxious or painful stimuli.

The testicles are roughly the size of a small egg. They are responsible for the development of sperm as well as the manufacture of the hormone testosterone. Behind the testicles sits the *epididymis*, a single coiled tube that is the site of sperm maturation and storage. The end of the epididymis results in a thick muscular tube, called the *vas deferens*, which carries sperm from the epididymis to the prostate to be ejaculated. The vas deferens is the most common site of sterility operations, or vasectomy.

The sperm is carried in the vas deferens to two structures that sit behind the prostate. These structures are called the *seminal vesicles*, glands roughly 2 inches in length that form a secretion which nourishes the sperm and which attach to the prostate as well. The prostate sits at the base of the bladder and creates a fluid that allows the nourishment and activation of sperm. The primary purpose of both the seminal vesicles and the prostate is to provide nourishment and a place for sperm to live before ejaculation. In fact, the majority of the ejaculate is composed of fluid from both these glands. A very small component, usually less than 5 percent, is actually spermatozoa, which is why the amount of ejaculate remains relatively unchanged after a vasectomy.

The prostate secretes the majority of the fluid. Two small glands sit just outside the diaphragm of the urogenital diaphragm, or the thick area that anchors the penis to the pubic bone. These structures, called the *bulbourethral glands*, produce a very small amount of clear fluid. This is the clear fluid that we see just prior to ejaculation. It may also contain very small amounts of spermatozoa as well.

Structural Abnormalities

One example of a structural problem is a bend to the penis. This bend may either be present at birth, termed *congenital*, or it may be acquired. We will discuss acquired bending in chapter 5 on Peyronie's disease. Most men have a slight bend or tilt to the penis. This is not considered abnormal. A bend is considered abnormal when it interferes with penetration. Rarely is a bend so substantial that a man is unable to penetrate. In this situation, a bend is generally in a downward position, with one corporal body longer than the other. When the bend is so severe that penetration is impossible, surgery is recommended. We will discuss this further in chapter 5.

Also, in 0.3 to 0.8 percent of male births, the urinary opening, or urethral meatus, lies farther back on the bottom of the shaft, a condition known as *hypospadias*. This by itself is not a significant problem, and surgery is only recommended if it is difficult to deposit semen into the vagina, or if it is difficult to urinate. There are many degrees of hypospadias, beginning from just below the tip of the penis, to well back to the base of the scrotum.

Another unusual anatomic condition includes the absence of testicles. Typically, for a man to be sexually functioning, the hormone testosterone must be circulating. One or both testicles must be present. When the testicles are not seen in the scrotum, they may be "undescended," or up inside the abdomen. This is a rare situation today because the condition is usually corrected shortly after birth.

The Physiology of Erections

I frequently use the analogy of achieving an erection to filling a tire with air. Achieving an erection takes air forced under pressure. More importantly, it takes an intact "tire" without a hole to maintain the air and allow it to expand. A defect in either of these two aspects will cause a "flat tire."

To achieve an erection, blood must enter the cavernosal artery and the artery then dilates in response to certain stimuli. The blood flow then increases, and when high blood flow enters the corporal body, the penis begins to engorge with blood. The tough membranes around the penis hold this in check to prevent uncontrolled expansion and make this a rigid structure. The smooth muscle inside the corporal body relaxes, allowing the spaces to dilate and trapping more blood in the penis based on the corporo-veno-occlusive mechanism. Again, this is the ability to maintain blood in the erect penis. The inside of the erect penis has relatively high pressures.

The key to the entire system is smooth muscle. The percent of smooth muscle dictates the ability to achieve and maintain erections. Roughly 45 percent of the cavernosal body is made up of smooth muscle. A whole cascade of hormonal events takes place to create an erection. While the exact details of this complicated cascade are certainly not within the scope of this book, it is clear that nitrogen oxide is the likely neuro-transmitter involved in achieving an erection. Nitrogen oxide stimulates cyclic GMP (guanosine monophosphate), which is a transmitter, and triggers this corporal smooth muscle to dilate. Increasing the amount of this neurotransmitter, or preventing its breakdown are two ways in which we can help to facilitate the creation and maintenance of an erection. Many new medications work specifically on this intercellular system of the penis to maintain the erection, and we will discuss this in chapter 10 on new treatments.

Ejaculation

Generally, an ejaculation is a reflex event of a highly limited length of time. It is representative of multiple levels of neural input. Ejaculation, from a nervous system standpoint, can happen in two ways. The first is purely from the central nervous system. An example would be a nocturnal emission, or wet dream. Nocturnal emissions are common in adolescence and in men who are not sexually active. They are the result of erotic stimuli in the absence of either masturbation or sexual intercourse. The second type is a combination of friction associated with input from the central nervous system. This is the typical ejaculation that men are most familiar with.

Ejaculation is divided into several events. Sexual stimulation and friction provide the impulses that go into the spinal cord and into the brain. The autonomic nervous system will stimulate the sympathetic nerves to cause contraction of the male accessory sexual organs including the vas deferens, prostate, and seminal vesicles. This results in a seminal emission, which is composed of the sperm and the seminal fluid from both the prostrate and seminal vesicles. This emission is deposited in the posterior urethra. The ejaculation occurs when there is contraction of the bulbocavernosus muscle propelling the semen out of the penis. The typical ejaculation is between 2 and 5 cc. Semen will normally turn into a gel and remain so for approximately thirty minutes. Following this, it then liquefies.

A basic understanding of the anatomy and physiology of the male genitourinary system provides a framework to begin building a basic understanding of sexual dysfunction. In the next chapter, much of the information that is obtained from a medical history relates directly to anatomy and physiology. When doctors use this information it facilitates our understanding of the treatments and options available as well as how to prevent loss of erections due to aging.

Chapter 2
Your Medical History

The first visit to a physician's office with the complaint of erectile dysfunction can be an unnerving experience. It is important to realize from the beginning that if you don't tell your physician exactly what is going on, there is no way that he or she is going to know the problem. In my own experience, patients will frequently come in for a minor, unrelated complaint and not reveal the true purpose of their visit until I specifically ask, "How are your erections?" Unfortunately, a medical professional's knowledge also comes from the same "textbooks" as everyone else's. Physicians uncomfortable with discussing erectile dysfunction may not pursue the appropriate line of questioning. This is often very frustrating for patients.

Most men, when asked in a straightforward, matter-of-fact manner will answer in a straightforward manner. But when the physician is uncomfortable in discussing this topic, he will tend to use confusing medical jargon and not lend himself to an open conversational style. Many physicians are poorly trained in sexual functioning. It is a myth that medical schools offer extensive courses on the subject. In fact, during medical school at the University of Virginia, part of my training included a "sex weekend," which basically consisted of watching pornographic movies for two days. These movies spanned every type of sexual practice from bestiality to group homosexuality and were followed by open discussions with groups of "alternative lifestyle" individuals. These were nothing more than graphic descriptions of unusual sexual practices. Although the purpose was to desensitize students to alternative sexual practices and make them more comfortable with taking a sexual history, in reality, students who had trouble dealing with sexual topics before the "sex weekend" never really learned to take an adequate sexual history and still had trouble dealing with sexual topics after the weekend.

Unfortunately, physicians as well as patients learn most of their sexual information from their peers, and sadly, much of this is not factual. What most patients don't realize is that they are consumers. If their questions are not being answered in a professional, comfortable fashion, they should seek advice from a physician who is comfortable speaking about this problem. It is perfectly normal to be uncomfortable about discussing a personal topic such as erectile dysfunction, but it should certainly not be embarrassing.

The discussion between doctor and patient frequently involves topics that have not even been shared with the

W.S., a fifty-year-old male, came to the office by himself. He had a substantial problem with both achieving and maintaining an erection for several years. After a careful historical review it became clear that he never actually asked his partner to have sexual intercourse. Throughout their relationship, when either partner desired intercourse they would use alternate terms for intercourse or pet names for their genitals. Anticipated sexual activity was termed, "having a date." In this man's history, he was allowed to have intercourse at a specific time and day each month. Unfortunately, if he was unable to achieve an erection at that moment, he was denied sex until the following month. His sexual partner would become very angry with him and frequently wouldn't speak to him for several days thereafter. He developed a pattern of severe premature ejaculation early on in the relationship, which was based completely upon his failure to communicate with his partner. It merely took an open discussion between him and his partner to alleviate the situation entirely.

patient's sexual partner. I'm always amazed by the number of men who are sexually frustrated but yet never come out and simply ask their partner if they can have sexual relations. Many men who seek help with this problem live with it for months, even years. It is human nature to think that a problem will go away and that by avoiding it we will not be confronted with its consequences. This underscores the problem that we as a society have in talking about the sensitive topics of sexual relationships, body image, and even illness.

The Initial Consultation

When preparing to go to a physician's office for the initial consultation, it is important to consider many things before the visit. The physician's office may or may not send you a questionnaire beforehand to help you put things into perspective. I currently use a questionnaire that generates a score and rates the severity of the erectile dysfunction. The International Index of Erectile Function Questionnaire (see appendix A) is an instrument for measuring male sexual dysfunction in a clinical setting. There are several questionnaires available, and many practices use a general questionnaire that reviews salient points on sexual drive, erections, and ejaculation, as well as the perception of sexual problems and overall satisfaction. The scoring system provides a means of measuring how severe the problem is and helps to put patients at ease. Then the physician and the patient can be on the same track when discussing erectile dysfunction. The questionnaire allows me to grade the erectile dysfunction from severe dysfunction to no dysfunction at all.

On the day of the consultation, it is also important to have the sexual partner present, if possible. This may not be practical if there are several partners and the sexual partner is uncomfortable talking about sexual problems outside the relationship.

Risk Factors

It is also important to review other general medical problems that may have an effect on erections, including medications and prior surgical procedures.

Another thing to think of when preparing for the initial consultation includes smoking history. Oftentimes I ask, "Do you smoke?" Patients will then tell me, "Oh, no, I quit." At this point I always ask when they quit and how long and how much they smoked. It is not surprising to find people replying, "Well, I quit last week." I still consider these patients smokers.

It is essential to bring a complete list of medications including the dosage that you are taking to the first office visit. Remember to mention all medicines including vitamins and herbal supplements. Many herbal supplements can have direct effects on genital tissues and can be associated with sexual dysfunction. Patients often do not realize the potency of these herbal compounds.

A patient's age is a key factor. Erectile dysfunction increases with age as revealed by the Massachusetts Male Aging Study.

I then discuss and characterize the quality of the patient's erections using a scale that rates erections from 0 to 10. A 10 is a perfect erection: rigid, the best erection ever. An erection that is barely able to penetrate is approximately a 5. When there is no swelling, or tumescence, of the penis whatsoever, this is a 0. Before the penis can become rigid, it becomes tumescent.

Libido is another component of the male sexual response. Problems with libido are usually related to depression, stress, partner dissatisfaction, and even hormonal imbalances. When asked about desire, men with erectile dysfunction will often respond by saying that they have no desire. What they really mean is that they are afraid to initiate sexual activity because of fear of failure. This is not a true loss of desire, but it is a good indicator of organic erectile dysfunction. The man who has lost all interest in sexual activity has a true loss of desire. He may get an erection, but he is not interested in pursuing sexual intercourse. This is an uncommon situation, and immediately indicates an unusual cause of erectile dysfunction called *prolactinoma*. This is a prolactin-secreting tumor that we will discuss extensively at a later point in chapter 4 on treatment. During a patient history, I also focus on the things that can affect erections including the timing of intercourse, masturbation, and the patient's work schedule.

Sexual Intercourse

At this point I always inquire when was the last time he had intercourse and how hard the penis was during intercourse. If the erection wasn't as hard as it could have been, I ask when was the last time it was rock-hard, an erection characterized as a 10. At this point, many men will have trouble characterizing their erections.

A simple, helpful tool to characterize an erection is to ask, "Could you hang a towel on it?" Although this sounds somewhat ridiculous, many men can relate to this. When describing a rock-hard erection, I often ask, "Could you hang a wet

M.F. was a forty-five-year-old man who presented the office with difficulty achieving and maintaining an erection. He came in at the urging of his wife. He had no risk factors and was otherwise a healthy vigorous male. He did indicate, however, that he had no difficulty with erectile dysfunction at all when he was with his girlfriend. This, of course, was given in a confidential nature, but it pointed to substantial marital distress and discord. This is not an uncommon scenario, so I always inquire how the patient's erections are with other partners.

towel on it?" This to me denotes a sufficient erection for penetration. I also try to determine the presence of morning erections and characterize their quality, again using the same 0 to 10 scale. Finally, I discuss whether the erection was the same with masturbation as with intercourse. This question can be somewhat uncomfortable for some men, but if asked in a professional manner, it is rarely a problem. It is not uncommon to find a situation where an erection will be very good with a partner's girlfriend and poor with the patient's wife. You'll never find this out if you don't ask.

One of the key things to ask in the medical history is, "Can you ejaculate with a soft penis?" This can be one of the most important indicators of an organic problem. I try to use the history to give me a feeling as to whether this is organic or has an underlying psychological problem. I also use the history to help guide me as to how aggressive a laboratory investigation and other subsequent tests need to be. When a problem is organic, medication or a concurrent

Z.F. was a forty-five-year-old man who presented the office with an inability to maintain his erection. He had an extremely physically intensive job, but his examination was entirely normal. He also had excellent desire and a supportive partner present. I performed a penile injection on the patient, and while the medication worked to produce what was a rock-hard erection, he actually fell asleep on the table. It became readily apparent after a careful history, that the man worked sixteen hours a day at heavy physical labor and was exhausted at the time of anticipated sexual relations. After we dealt with this problem, he was able to restore his erectile functioning and found he performed much better after he had a good night's sleep. Reworking his schedule produced dramatic results.

medical condition can be an obvious cause. Years ago, the majority of erectile dysfunction cases were diagnosed as psychological. More recently, however, with more sensitive tools and measurements of erections, we now know that this is not true, and in fact, the vast majority of erections are organic in nature.

Ejaculation

I then discuss ejaculation—when it happens, how long the patient is able to maintain penetration before the ejaculation happens, how much ejaculate is produced, and whether it is a whitish color, which is considered normal, or more rarely, stained with blood. Some men will say they don't know, but I tell them that the only way to know is to look. Many men, however, will know the volume of ejaculate because they have a feeling for how much comes out at the time of masturbation.

Blood in the ejaculate is usually the result of a simple infection. This condition, termed *hematospermia*, is easily treated, and reassurance is the most important prescription in this situation.

Related Causes and Conditions

Medications

Discussion of a medical history usually includes allergies to medications as well as seasonal allergies. Many men will self-treat with decongestants which contain drugs that can cause the early loss of erections and retard ejaculations. Drugs that are nasal-drying agents are frequently used during cough and cold season. Classically, we have used cousins of these drugs to prevent erections and to help treat a painful condition known as *priapism*. (We will discuss this extensively in chapter 5.) Review of the medications is extremely important. The difficulty with evaluating drug effects on erections lies in the fact that some drugs associated with erections are also associated with impotence, erectile dysfunction, and at the same time, can be associated with causing an erection to not go away.

The Massachusetts Male Aging Study found that

complete loss of erections was more significant in men who were taking medications and particularly medications to treat diabetes, high blood pressure, and cardiac problems. Drugs used to treat hypertension include diuretics, and particularly thiazide diuretics, the mainstay of diuretics in the United States. Numerous studies report diuretics to be associated with erectile dysfunction. The diuretic spironolactone has been strongly associated with erectile dysfunction and has also been associated with decreased libido and the development of breasts in men, a condition termed *gynecomastia*. Drugs used to treat high blood pressure include alpha-blocking agents, such as prazosin. This drug, in addition to being related to loss of erections, has also been related to an erection that won't go away, or priapism.

The beta-blocking agents, which are also used to treat high blood pressure, have also been strongly associated with loss of erection. These drugs include propranolol and atenolol. Other drugs used to treat high blood pressure include methyldopa, an older blood pressure medication that has been strongly related to erectile dysfunction, and the ACE (angiotensin converting enzyme) inhibitors, which include captopril. These have been associated with erectile dysfunction, though not as strongly. In my experience, the problem with identifying a drug that may be causing erectile dysfunction is that it is usually not reasonable to change the medication. Rather, using another medication to treat the erectile dysfunction along with one of the various therapeutic options currently available is usually a better option.

In patients with arthritis, it has been postulated that the chronic use of aspirin and ibuprofen, by their effect on decreasing prostaglandins, can actually result in sexual dys-

F.D. was a seventy-one-year-old man presenting to the office with painful, swollen breasts, and a sudden loss of erections. He had no identifiable cause, and a careful history and physical examination identified that his wife recently began using hormone cream. During intercourse, he actually absorbed some of this cream through his penis. We successfully reduced this absorption by instituting the use of a condom. This resolved the problem within one month.

function. Clinically, we do see an increase in erectile dysfunction in patients with arthritis. While not proven, this certainly is an attractive hypothesis.

Many of the drugs used to treat psychiatric conditions have a strong effect on loss of erections. These drugs include thioridazine, which in addition to causing erectile dysfunction can also prevent ejaculation. Many antidepressants have been strongly associated with a decrease in libido and erectile dysfunction as well. Some of the other drugs that can cause problems include cimetidine, which causes a decreased libido and erectile dysfunction in up to 50 percent of cases, and ranitidine, which can also produce a loss of libido and erectile failure but certainly much less so than with cimetidine. The heart medication digoxin has shown a substantial association with loss of erections because it causes an increased level of estrogen and decreased level of testosterone. Digoxin has been proposed as a drug to help treat erections that won't go away. Other drugs include the drug finasteride, used to treat prostate enlargement, which not only can affect erections but decreases the volume of ejaculate as well. Finally, alcohol, marijuana, and a whole host of other drugs can actually affect erections.

I have also encountered several cases of men who have intercourse with women who, because of vaginal dryness, use hormone creams. During intercourse they absorb the estrogen through their penis, resulting in breast enlargement and a loss of erections. This is another good reason to have the patient's partner present when taking a sexual history.

Prior Medical Conditions

I also inquire about prior surgical procedures. I especially focus on procedures that affect the genitourinary tract such as a radical prostatectomy. This procedure is rapidly becoming one of the most commonly performed operations in the United States for the treatment of prostate cancer. As a consequence of this operation, erectile dysfunction has become more common and probably affects two-thirds of these men. Childhood surgeries may also have an effect on the testicles. Prior bladder surgeries that may have been performed in childhood can affect the ability to ejaculate normally.

When discussing prior medical problems, we focus extensively on high blood pressure, diabetes, heart disease, gout, and arthritis, all of which have been implicated in making erectile dysfunction worse, both either from the disease state or from the medications used to treat them. Prior childhood illnesses such as mumps are also relevant. When mumps is contracted after puberty, it can damage the testicles to the point that they become small and shrunken and fail to produce adequate male hormones.

Personal Habits

Personal habits include the patient's smoking history: the types of products smoked, frequency, and time length. When talking about cigars and pipes it is important to characterize the amount smoked. A good way to characterize this in pipe smokers is the number of pouches used per week, or the number of pipe bowls per week. And it is not infrequent to find a pipe or cigar smoker who inhales.

Alcohol consumption is also part of the patient's medical history. Heavy alcohol consumption is considered to be more than one case of beer per week or its equivalent. Although this seems dramatic by some standards, many people have several drinks each evening and yet they correlate this habit the least with sexual dysfunction. For the purposes of erectile dysfunction, I consider the amount of alcohol consumed excessive when it has a deleterious effect on erections. For example, the consumption of a case of beer a day would be a significant finding in a patient with erectile dysfunction.

Chronic marijuana usage is well documented to result in erectile dysfunction and infertility. A doctor should also discuss cocaine and other drug usage, including the use of anabolic steroids. Men will not usually volunteer this type of information unless specifically asked.

B.F. was a fifty-five-year-old man who presented with erectile dysfunction. He had an approximate two-year history of an inability to achieve and maintain an erection. He brought his wife to the consultation. At the initial stage of the interview, it was noted that she became hostile and frequently interrupted the examiner, asking why she needed to be there. She remained extremely hostile during the interview, both verbally and nonverbally. When asked what she wanted from this interview, she stated that she "didn't care if it ever worked again." She got up and left angry in the middle of the interview. B.F. looked up and said, "Now you see the problem." After a careful physical examination, I felt this was a combination of both an organic and a psychological problem. At the time of the interview, after the partner left, the patient related to me that he was unable to maintain an erection, even during masturbation. This to me was more indicative of an organic problem. This factor, however, was greatly overshadowed by a psychological problem, specifically his partner, who for a variety of reasons had absolutely no interest in sexual relations or intimacy. My recommendation was to return after the marital conflict was resolved. Although it was quite possible to restore sexual functioning, this man's situation would probably have not allowed this.

Family History

The next topic of discussion is the family history. Basic overall health can be traced through a family tree. As we learn more about family dynamics, the old adage "You can't choose your parents" rings true. Many cardiovascular and cancer-related deaths are frequently traceable to family history. Even Peyronie's disease can be a familial disease in some instances, so I always inquire about it. It is unusual, however, for patients to know whether or not there is a family history of Peyronie's disease. Many men are not aware that their father had a problem with erectile dysfunction. But every now and then I am surprised to find that some men are able to describe their father's erections in detail. This tells me that their relationship is open enough for them to talk about it.

Take-Home Points

- It is essential to go to the consultation with as much information available as possible.

- Bring your sexual partner with you when feasible.

- If you are unhappy in any way with the line of questioning or with the physician's manner in attempting to gain the history, seek advice elsewhere.

- Always attempt to go to the medical professional that has the most training in his or her field.

- If a physician fails to take an adequate history, find another physician.

- If a physician does not answer questions to your satisfaction, find another physician.

- Bring a list of all medications you are taking, including over-the-counter medications as well as herbal medications.

Chapter 3

The Physical Examination

The sexual physical examination begins the moment you walk into the physician's office. From the time you fill out the basic information for the chart to the time that you enter the examination room, your physician should notice subtle things. This includes the following observations about the patient's appearance:

- Is there normal musculature and stature? In other words, does the patient have the appropriate amount of muscles for his age, or is he generally extremely thin or extremely well-muscled? (An overly muscular stature sometimes indicates the use of anabolic steroids.)

- Is there obesity? If so, to what degree?

- Are there any obvious spinal or nerve problems? This can be readily observed by the patient's gait.

- Is there difficulty walking?

- Is there an obvious drooping or paralysis of an extremity? This may indicate a previous stroke.

These things are evident on casual observation as so much of medical practice is nothing more than observation and common sense.

Physical Appearance

Stature

Stature can be categorized into three basic body types: ectomorph—the tall, thin, male with minimal body fat; mesomorph—a far more common body type with average appearance and maybe some thickening at the waistline, but generally the waist is narrower than the shoulders; and endomorph—the individual whose waist is far wider than the shoulders.

Hormonal Attributes

I also look at the amount of facial and body hair present. Generally, a man with sparse facial hair who doesn't shave frequently may have a hormonal problem. Male pattern baldness, contrary to the popular belief, does not usually relate to the amount of circulating male hormone.

Next, I check the blood pressure. Many times the blood pressure will be elevated just because of the stress of being in the medical office. While examining the patient's genitals, I first look at the secondary sexual characteristics. What this means is, how much pubic hair is present? The pattern of the pubic hair is termed the escutcheon. In females, the pubic hair usually does not form a line toward the umbilicus as it does in males.

I examine the chest for evidence of breast enlargement or nipple discharge. Both these problems can point to medication side effects or an abnormal hormonal system. I also look at the amount of chest hair present.

I examine the abdomen for evidence of masses such as lumps or fatty tumors. I carefully look at the skin of the chest for evidence of skin lesions. Spider angiomas are commonly discovered at this point. These are small, red skin lesions that have the appearance of tiny spiders and are frequently found on the abdomen. This generally suggests chronic liver disease, a common cause of erectile dysfunction.

Genital Examination

It is not uncommon for patients to feel uncomfortable during this portion of the exam. It can be embarrassing to have your genitals examined in a way that you probably wouldn't do yourself, and it may be uncomfortable to be in a position with your pants and underwear pulled down. As a physician I try to do this examination as quickly as possible to minimize exposure of the genitals, and I always wear gloves when examining patients. If your physician fails to

P.A. was an elderly gentleman who presented for an examination. His scrotum was so elongated that when he went to have a bowel movement, it actually dropped in the water of the toilet. It was such a distressing problem for him that one of his testicles had to be removed in order to prevent this from happening. This is an extreme example of an abnormally long scrotum.

wear gloves when examining your genitals, you should ask him to do so. This is similar to a dentist examining your mouth without a glove, or a gynecologist not wearing gloves. It is inappropriate.

When checking the groin I look for evidence of bulges that can indicate hernias. I then feel the spermatic cords. These are the structures that carry blood to and from the testes and that also contain the tube called the vas deferens.

I then examine the testicles. It is important to note their size and any adjacent structures. Testicles are roughly 4 cm in length and approximately the size of a small egg. They should be smooth and their examination should not be tremendously uncomfortable.

At this point I try to teach the patient what some of the other lumps and bumps of the scrotum are. This way, the patient can familiarize himself with what is a normal finding and what is abnormal. I always show the patient what a normal testicle examination should be like, and I strongly encourage monthly self-examinations.

I then examine the scrotum for evidence of rashes or infections. Scrotal skin is typically hair bearing, and depending upon the temperature of the room, may be contracted or relaxed. In some older men, the scrotum may be so relaxed that it almost hangs down to the level of the kneecaps. I recommend tighter underwear for men whose scrotums hang very low.

Long-term usage of boxer shorts tends to produce more problems with the scrotum with rubbing on the inner side of the thighs. The structures behind the testicles called the *epididymis*, a single coiled tube that carries sperm from the testicles to the vas deferens, are a frequent site of inflammation and enlargement. A cystic enlargement of this area in which fluid may be trapped and then stored is known as a *spermatocele*. Spermatoceles may become extremely large in size. I check the scrotum for the presence of small cystic structures called *sebaceous cysts*. These cysts have a waxy appearance, and they become inflamed and drain a cheesy material.

Additionally, fluid may collect around the testicle itself. This fluid collection is known as a *hydrocele*, which is distinct from the spermatocele. The difference lies in the position. A spermatocele usually sits above and behind a testicle, whereas a hydrocele lies in front of and encompasses the entire testicle. The hydrocele fluid collection can become massive, and its size alone can not only be a cause of embarrassment, but a physical impediment to intercourse by causing concealment of the penis.

If left untreated, fluid collections in the scrotum can come close to the size of basketballs and totally conceal the penis. I see this at least once or twice a month in my practice. These men, for a variety of reasons, will choose to live with this problem and avoid sexual intercourse. This condition is completely treatable by a simple surgical procedure, and it should not be an impediment to satisfactory sexual intercourse.

Testicles that are poorly developed or have been damaged may be a consequence of either testicle surgery or damage during vasectomy. More commonly this is the result of a mumps infection. Small testicles are termed *atrophic*. They can frequently be poor producers of testosterone.

If the penis is uncircumcised, I check whether the foreskin easily pulls up and back on the glans. If the skin is tight and it is not possible to pull the foreskin back, this is a condition called *phimosis*. Phimosis makes it extremely painful to get an erection and may be the cause of erectile dysfunction in some instances. I pull the foreskin back and examine the moist inner side of the foreskin for lesions, such as early cancers or venereal warts. Small firm bumps on the rim of the head of the penis, known as the corona, are *hirsutoid papillomas*. This upsets many men who believe that this is a venereal disease, but they are quite common. Men who examine their penis can identify the location and duration of many of the small bumps and whether they have been present their entire lives.

I inquire about any discoloration or small birthmarks on the penis itself and how long the mole or discoloration has been present. Any mole that changes color or consistency or bleeds easily needs to be biopsied.

I next examine the urethral meatus, the opening where the urine comes out at the tip of the penis. I check its size and evaluate to see if it has been narrowed or scarred. I always make sure that I can retract both edges and examine the inside of the urethra since this is a common site for venereal warts and discharges from sexually transmitted diseases.

An infection on the head of the penis is known as *balanitis*. The most common cause of balanitis is a yeast infection. This is prevalent in men with diabetes due to the high concentration of sugar in the urine that promotes the growth of yeast under the foreskin causing infection. Balanitis can also be transmitted from a sexual partner who has a yeast infection. It is generally painful and is treated with topical creams to prevent infection. If the creams do not get rid of the infection, then a procedure known as a *circumcision* is performed in which the outer foreskin that covers the head of the penis is cut. Circumcision was once a common operation in newborn babies, but it is being performed less often because of concerns that it is painful for the infant.

I also gently pull on the penis to see how mobile it is. Certain scarring conditions can cause the penis to be rigid and not allow it to be pulled in a gentle fashion. I feel the shaft of the penis for evidence of Peyronie's plaques and evaluate whether the superficial veins have become fibrotic or cordlike. These cords always run in a vertical fashion on the penis instead of around the penis. Any changes are usually the consequence of minor trauma during sexual intercourse.

An optional part of the physical examination is to test the sensation of the glans penis. The head of the penis has a number of receptors for increased sensation or sensitivity. Most men don't realize that the majority of sensation of their penis is actually on the glans. The shaft of the penis has relatively few receptors for sensation. The uncircumcised head of the penis is generally much more sensitive because the head is always covered by foreskin. This prevents it from chronic rubbing on clothing and dulling of the sensation.

The final part of the external exam is to feel the area

between the rectum and the scrotum known as the *perineum*. In doing so, I am looking for infected cysts, lesions, or draining sinuses. A draining sinus is an area that drains from the rectum outside the anus to an area in the perineum. This is a condition that may be seen with certain inflammatory diseases of the bowel and can be an extremely painful situation.

The DRE

A digital rectal examination involves inserting a gloved lubricated finger in the rectum to check not only the tone of the rectum and anus but also the prostate and for the presence of any other rectal or anal lesions.

There should be sufficient tone in the rectum so that it is tight around the examiner's finger. Decreased tone indicates either a neurologic problem or a situation where the rectum is chronically dilated, a result of anal intercourse or chronic insertion of foreign bodies into the rectum. Sometimes the anal sphincter is so tight that digital penetration is not possible. This is either a consequence of being unable to relax during the examination or a result of a spinal condition or nerve damage. The reflex known as the *bulbocavernosus reflex* is elicited by squeezing the head of the penis briskly with the finger and causing the anal sphincter to contract suddenly around the finger in the rectum. It is generally quite noticeable. *Hyperreflexia*, or an abnormal bulbocavernosus reflex, generally occurs from certain nervous conditions such as multiple sclerosis. Hyperreflexia

E.B. was a twenty-nine-year-old man brought by his wife because of decreased sexual desire. History indicated that he had mumps as a teenager and that he had never really been sexually active or interested in sex. Upon examination, he was found to have sparse facial and body hair and a normal-sized penis, however, both testes were smaller than peas. In this situation, the diagnosis of mumps orchitis was made. Treatment with testosterone replacement showed dramatic results.

refers to reflexes that are much more vigorous than normal. For instance, if you tap your knee, your foot will reflexively kick outward. Hyperreflexia means that the foot kicks out much higher and faster than normal.

I also evaluate for the presence or absence of stool in the rectum. Chronic constipation can cause the rectum to be extremely dilated resulting in blockage, or fecal impaction. Hemorrhoids are also detectable at this point, both external and internal. Patients who have had prior surgery to the anus may have scarring or strictures that prevent rectal examination.

An examination of the prostate includes all areas of the prostate. In thin individuals, I am frequently able to feel the top of the prostate in the area called the *seminal vesicles*. If this area is inflamed, the ejaculate may be bloody, a condition known as *seminal vesiculitis*.

I then feel the blood vessels in the groin, including the major artery that runs from the groin to the legs called the *femoral artery*. A decreased pulse in this area may be an important clue that there is decreased blood flow to the bottom half of the body. This finding may also be an indication as to the cause of erectile dysfunction. Examination of the legs often reveals evidence of severe diabetes or decreased blood flow. These are also important clues in the workup of erectile dysfunction.

Remember, the physical examination is extremely important and should complement the medical history. It is important that the physical examination be complete. If the physician fails to examine the prostate or does only a cursory examination, then obtain another opinion.

Penis Size

One of the most common questions patients ask me is, "What is a normal-sized penis?" There really is no consensus on how to measure the penis, but generally speaking, an adequate penis is defined as one that allows penetration of the vagina sufficient enough to permit fertilization and the ability to stand upright to urinate. When these two criteria are met, the penis is an adequate size.

A flaccid and an erect penis differ tremendously in length. Measurement of a flaccid penis is not a good predictor of the length of an erect penis. Actual penile length measurement should be made with a full erection with a rigid ruler starting at the top of the penis between the tip to the point where the penis anchors the body at the bone, called the *symphysis pubis*. It is extremely important not to include the foreskin, especially in men who have elongated droopy foreskin. It is also important to avoid as much of the superficial fat as possible.

P.F. was brought by his wife for evaluation of potential erectile dysfunction. The patient's wife was a registered nurse who reported that her husband had good desire but difficulty completing the act of intercourse. Physical examination disclosed a congenital abnormality of the penis where the urinary opening actually opened toward the base of the penis, a condition called *hypospadias*. When he achieved an erection, it was so bent that it precluded adequate vaginal penetration. The situation was easily remedied by surgery. Interestingly, the patient's wife had seen numerous normal penises as a nurse. They had been married several years before this condition became a problem and vaginal penetration was not part of their lovemaking. Apparently, she was now interested in becoming pregnant, which was what precipitated the visit to the clinic.

Studies show that the typical erection is roughly 5 inches in length, and I would certainly concur with this in my own busy urologic practice. The amount of body fat dictates the length of the penis as well. A general rule of thumb is that for every 30 pounds over ideal body weight, one can generally expect to lose an inch of penis size. The penis does not actually shrink, but more of it is concealed under a layer of fat. The more fat that surrounds the base of the penis, the less that length is apparent. While it is unusual to see a very large penis on an obese man, it is also true that a short penis can look quite long on an extremely thin man. (We will discuss penile-lengthening procedures more extensively in chapter 9.)

I look at the physical examination as a "blue light special." It allows me the opportunity to do a complete physical examination of a man who probably otherwise would never get a complete physical.

A careful history and physical examination is essential in determining the etiology of the erectile dysfunction. Laboratory tests should only be performed when the history and physical examination determine the need for these. In the next chapter, we will discuss the appropriate laboratory workup of erectile dysfunction.

Take-Home Points

- A complete physical examination is essential to determine the etiology of erectile dysfunction.

- The digital rectal examination is an important aspect of the exam.

- If the physician does not examine you thoroughly, find another physician.

- The physical examination is an excellent time to learn how to perform a testicular self-examination.

- Examine your testicles monthly for early testicular cancers.

Chapter 4

Diagnosing Erectile Dysfunction

Laboratory Investigation

After a careful and thorough history and physical examination, I generally tailor the use of laboratory investigation to the individual patient. I try to avoid doing every lab to every patient as it is typically a waste of money.

Urinalysis

The initial lab procedure, the urinalysis, is an inexpensive test that is done by the treating physician in the office. It provides a wealth of information. The urinalysis provides the most medical information in the most cost-efficient way. This test will provide information regarding the presence or absence of infection, as well as the possibility of diabetes.

I frequently make the initial diagnosis of diabetes when evaluating men for sexual dysfunction. Diabetes is one of the major causes of erectile dysfunction in the United States. I am also able to screen for urologic problems such as blood in the urine, which can be a prognostic sign of cancer, and make a positive impact on the patient's life by finding a cancer that would otherwise not be discovered until it had spread. We also frequently find urinary tract infections by examining the urine during this phase of the investigation. Following a careful urinalysis, the remainder of the tests should be at the discretion of the physician, based on suspicious findings in the history or physical examination.

Testosterone Level

The next test I consider is the testosterone level. Low serum testosterone can be a cause of erectile dysfunction. Truly low serum testosterone level is indicated by the history and physical examination, including decreased sex drive, poor erections, dry skin, small testicles, a decreased need to shave, and a decreased amount of muscle mass.

The single best test for testosterone level is the free serum testosterone. Free and total testosterone means the amount of testosterone that is active in the body. By measuring the free testosterone, you are measuring the type of testosterone that is the most active in the patient. Remember that the testosterone is transported through the body bound to a substance that helps carry it through the various organs requiring it for growth.

The vast majority of men who have their testosterone checked only have a total testosterone level. This can be adequate in most cases, but if there is any question as to whether the testosterone is truly low, I do a free serum testosterone test. Men with lower levels of binding globulin, which can artificially lower the testosterone, include older men and men on low-fat diets or those with liver damage or who are taking other hormones that compete for these binding sites. Men who have very high levels of the binding globulin include obese men and men on high-fat diets. A truly low free testosterone level finding should always be repeated to be certain of the diagnosis prior to placing a patient on what may be lifelong therapy. The treatment for low serum testosterone is androgen replacement therapy, which is not without side effects. We will discuss this extensively in chapter 6.

Serum Prolactin Level

The next test I generally obtain in certain clinical situations is a serum prolactin level. A normal testosterone level rarely accompanies an elevated prolactin level in men. Common causes of a mildly elevated prolactin level include diabetes, kidney failure, and certain medications such as alphamethyldopa, female hormones, and the antipsychotic drugs, phenothiazines. The instance of elevated prolactin is extremely rare, although it is one of the most common forms of pituitary hormone excesses.

Clinically, cases of truly elevated prolactin levels can be predicted from the clinical history. The key question in the clinical history is to ask about a lack of interest versus an inability to get an erection. These men will typically say that they are able to get a good erection, but they have no interest in having sexual relations.

When a prolactin-secreting tumor, which is a benign tumor, enlarges, it can put pressure on the optic nerves causing visual changes. It is also not uncommon to see headaches and breast swelling in these men. When an elevated prolactin level is found, it is extremely important for the physician to rule out other tumors as a cause. This is a fairly straightforward workup and merely requires a CAT scan or MRI of the pituitary area. A CAT scan is an X ray that looks at the area of the pituitary gland where prolactin-secreting tumors can grow. Interestingly, as the prolactin level gets higher, the chances of finding an abnormal pituitary on an X ray increase dramatically. This is an extremely easy problem to treat with simple oral medications.

Gonadotropins

Other laboratory tests in the evaluation of erectile dysfunction include the gonadotropins. Gonadotropins are substances produced by the pituitary gland that are useful when trying to discover the reasons for low testosterone levels. The first clinically useful test is called the luteinizing hormone, the hormone that stimulates the production of testosterone. A man with low testosterone and a low luteinizing hormone (LH) is diagnosed as *hypogonadotrophic*. The condition called hypogonadism is low testosterone and a high LH, which indicates testicular failure.

Thyroid Function

A thyroid function test may be done in situations where the man may have a low thyroid level. This can generally be associated with a decrease in sexual drive and weight gain.

Lipid Profile

More frequently, I will check the lipid profile, which is a measure of the cholesterol level as well as the components of cholesterol, known as high-density lipoproteins and low-density lipoproteins. One of the startling facts revealed by the Massachusetts Male Aging Study is that men with erectile dysfunction frequently have low levels of high-density lipoproteins, the good form of cholesterol. Men with high levels of cholesterol and triglycerides, which are a form of fat in the bloodstream, frequently have erectile dysfunction directly related to this condition.

Blood Count

In certain situations, a complete blood count and chemistry profile is necessary, especially among men who indicate other, more unusual causes. A man who has evidence of liver disease or alcoholism should have a liver function test, as this can directly affect the ability to achieve an erection. Renal function tests should be done in men who also indicate renal failure. A blood count, which measures the amount of red blood cells in the bloodstream, can be useful in determining anemia as the cause of erectile dysfunction. Some men are so anemic that they are extremely fatigued, which is apparent in a physical examination. Some physicians may want to order every test on every patient. Remember, this is unnecessary and costly, and generally does not improve the patient in any way.

Other Investigations

Penile Biothesiometry

One useful way to evaluate the nerves that carry sensation away from the penis is by the use of a technique called penile biothesiometry. This is a quantitative measure of the vibratory sense of the penis. A biothesiometer consists of a device that vibrates at a known frequency, and it is compared to other parts of the body with known vibration thresholds. This tends to become less reliable in older patients because as men age they tend to lose sensation. Still, it is a reasonable, cost-effective test.

The device is placed on the tip of the finger, and slowly the frequency is increased until the vibration is felt. This is then used as a baseline to compare the vibration sense of the penis as well. It is a useful way to detect early neuropathic disease in younger men, particularly in men with diabetes. It is also used in men who have had circumcisions and complain that the head of the penis has lost sensation.

Duplex Ultrasound

The Duplex ultrasound is a relatively new procedure and probably the single best test to evaluate male erectile dysfunction. Duplex ultrasound combined with an intercavernosal injection has pretty much replaced all other tests that are currently available. This single test can evaluate both the early and late stages of an erection, as well as venous leakage. The technique utilizes a special Doppler ultrasound device that uses a color-type system which assesses the blood flow direction and provides a way to evaluate the volume of flow into and out of the penis.

The technique is fairly simple. It is done by first taking a picture of the flaccid penis. We include the corporal bodies and the spongiosum, which is the spongy layer that surrounds the urethra. There we look for dense areas that may represent Peyronie's disease. We also look for calcifications that can indicate scarring or early blood vessel changes consistent with atherosclerosis. We then induce an erection by injecting prostaglandin. We repeat the study at one-, five-, and fifteen-minute intervals. Using this technique, we are able to image the cavernosal arteries. We measure them both before and after the injection. If the patient responds poorly to this, we sometimes have the patient perform self-stimulation in order to take out of the equation any results of anxiety or embarrassment that may cause a loss of erection and confuse the results.

We are then able to evaluate patients who have arterial disease. Poor arterial dilation indicates poor blood flow in response to the injection. This is compared to data on the normal peak flow velocity and how fast the blood pressure should rise in the artery supplying blood to the penis. We are also able to visually evaluate the erection and document venous leakage. Persistently elevated diastolic flow correlates with venous leakage. Physicians not experienced in performing the tests and interpreting the data should not do these studies.

The blood flow test is particularly useful in patients with Peyronie's disease because it not only assesses how much blood flow is present, but how much bending there is and the presence of other lesions. I generally recommend this test on all patients who are undergoing a penile implant or corrective surgery. This provides good factual information to work with prior to proceeding with the surgical procedure.

Arteriography

Selective arteriography is recommended only for men who are candidates for arterial revasculization. These are usually young, healthy men who have suffered trauma to the penis or to the area under the scrotum known as the *perineum*. Prior to proceeding with an arteriogram, which is a very invasive procedure, a Duplex Doppler examination showing the presence of poor blood flow and indicating a probable arterial lesion should be performed. If an obstruction is visualized, it is important to document whether there is flow back through the blockage to the point of obstruction so that the patient will be sure to benefit from the procedure.

Microsurgical penile revascularization is an invasive procedure that should only be done in referral centers by experienced physicians. This is not an operation that most urologists do on a regular basis. The procedure performed is generally a microvascular arterial bypass. The objective of the surgery is to increase the blood flow to the corporal body and therefore improve the erections. The best candidates for surgery are men who have poor erections with spontaneous erections absent and in whom all studies indicate a pure arterial component. Patients with other diseases such as diabetes or heavy smokers are poor candidates for this type of operation.

Ideally, arterial surgery should be the way to treat erectile dysfunction since it seems logical that a damaged or blocked artery could easily be bypassed to provide the necessary blood needed to maintain an erection. Unfortunately, this is not the case because the patients who have this distinct arterial lesion are very limited.

Many physicians have spent a lot of time trying to develop an arterial bypass that can improve this condition, and numerous procedures have been developed. Patients who undergo arteriography should be highly motivated and have a complete workup to rule out all other causes of erectile dysfunction, including hormonal problems or venous leaks. Patients should not proceed with arteriography unless they are good candidates for revascularization.

Venous Leakage

Venous leakage is a relatively common cause of erectile dysfunction. An inability to achieve and maintain the full erection occurs because blood leaks out in the presence of an adequate arterial inflow due to a damaged veno-corporo-occlusive mechanism. There are five theorized types of venogenic impotence.

Type 1 is due to the presence of an excessively large number of veins exiting the corporal body. This is probably congenital and is seen in young men with primary erectile dysfunction.

Type 2 is the weakening of the tough outer membrane of the corporal membrane of the corporal body known as the *tunica albuginea*, resulting in poor compression of the veins, such as in elderly men. I consider this a wear-and-tear phenomenon.

Type 3 is the loss of compliance of the cavernosal smooth muscle because of Peyronie's disease or scarring degeneration in patients with severe hardening of the arteries.

Type 4 is poor relaxation of the cavernous smooth muscle due to inadequate release of the hormones it takes to create an erection. This is typically common in heavy smokers.

Type 5 results from abnormal communications between the corpora cavernosa and the spongiosum due to trauma or a prior procedure to treat priapism.

Patients with pure erectile dysfunction on the basis of a venous leak are rare, but many men have venous leakage as a component of their erectile dysfunction. Many years ago, we felt that this was a major problem, and during the early 1980s a great deal of venous leakage surgery was performed. We found that patients with specific venous leakage due to congenital abnormalities or specific trauma type situations do well with these types of operations, but the majority of patients do poorly. We still feel the first choice for patients who have venous leakage is a vacuum erection device or treatment with intercavernosal injections. The only patients who are candidates for a venous leakage operation are patients who have failed simple, noninvasive treatments.

Many people have attempted surgery for venous leakage. A host of different procedures attempt to make the diagnosis. All these techniques basically try to measure the pressures required to make blood leak out of the corporal bodies. Cavernosography is the technique of injecting dye into the corporal body to identify a leaking blood vessel. Prostaglandin is first injected to create an erection and then dye, which potentially identifies the site of the leakage. The results of these diagnostic procedures have not been dramatic.

When it has been determined that the patient is a good candidate for repair, the idea of treatment is to find the vein that is the source of the leakage and then tie it off. If the leaking vessel is near the base of the body, then an incision is made over that area. We feel that good candidates for venous surgery are those who have identified a localized leak and who have had a complete workup to rule out all the obvious causes for erectile dysfunction, including the Duplex Doppler examination. Surgical candidates should be non-smokers, young, and have no other medical problems. A preoperative X-ray examination called the *cavernosogram* should identify the site of the leaking vessel.

The complications with this type of operation are numerous, as with all operations. They include numbness of the penis, scarring, a shortening or twisting of the penis, and painful erections.

Dynamic Infusion Cavernosometry and Cavernosography

Dynamic infusion cavernosometry is a technique in which fluid is pumped into the penis at a known rate and pressure. This procedure helps us to define the veno-occlusive function during an erection. To do this test we administer prostaglandin E-1. We measure the rate of infusion required to get a rigid erection and then use this to help find how severe the venous leak is. As an adjunct to this procedure, we then instill contrast material, and this is termed a cavernosogram. We then use X rays to measure and to visualize any leaking vessels. This is particularly applicable in men who have Type 1 or Type 5 venous leaks.

Nocturnal Penile Tumescence Testing

Nocturnal penile erections have been associated with rapid eye movement (REM) sleep. Nocturnal penile tumescence (NPT) helps maintain erections by providing oxygenation to the penis. During REM sleep, men normally have several erections each night, each one lasting up to an hour. Thus, during the erection, the corporal bodies are exposed to the same oxygen level that the rest of the body experiences for up to four hours per day. In men who have poor penile blood flow, and therefore poor erections, this does not occur, hastening the development of scar tissue and loss of corporal smooth muscle. Therefore, nocturnal erections are extremely important for the maintenance of good erectile functioning. As men age, these episodes become fewer and shorter. Nocturnal penile tumescence monitoring is useful in patients who report a complete absence of erections but in whom a psychological component is suspected.

Before the advent of the newer techniques using the rigiscan, physicians used the postage stamp test. Basically, a series of stamps was placed around the base of the penis. If the patient awoke the next morning with the stamps unbroken, this indicated an organic problem. However, if the stamps were broken, this was felt to be a psychological problem. Following the postage stamp test was the development of the snap gauge, a Velcro band placed around the base of the penis that had three colored plastic film elements. Each film ruptured at a specific known force. It took 10 ounces of radial force to rupture the blue tab, 15 ounces to rupture the red tab, and 20 ounces to rupture the clear tab. These snap gauge results were reasonable. However, there was no way to measure rigidity. When the criteria for the snap gauge was carefully examined, it was found that half the men who broke two to three films actually had no rigidity by visual inspection. Because of this, it has lost some favor and it has been mostly supplanted by the rigiscan.

The rigiscan allows us to measure continuous tumescence monitoring, but it also provides rigidity information during the times when the patient is achieving an erection. In addition, it gives detailed information about how often the erections occur, for what period of time, and the rigidity and change in diameter. Rigidity is measured by placing a loop around the base of the penis, which is tightened every thirty seconds with a force of 2.8 Newtons. It records three sessions, and then it is downloaded into a computer. The newest version of the rigiscan uses software that can calculate an entire evening of tumescence and rigidity data into rigidity activity units and tumescence activity units. Several different types of patterns are measured by the rigiscan, including dissociation which is seen with Peyronie's disease. This pattern shows how the base of the penis gets hard and the tip past the areas of the Peyronie's plaque has poor rigidity and tumescence. Another pattern, termed uncoupling, occurs when there is good tumescence on both the base and tip, but poor rigidity. While rigiscan testing doesn't give an exact diagnosis, it can be extremely useful.

NPT studies are not perfect. Some problems, including sleep disorders and depression, can cause abnormal readings. This should be recognized when performing the study. Testing prior to surgery demonstrates that the patient does indeed have erectile dysfunction. If the patient has complications or needs surgery, such as repairing the implant, testing protects the patient against cases in which an insurance company attempts to avoid payment for a service and in medical malpractice. An NPT study supports the urologist's diagnosis of erectile dysfunction.

It is important to tailor the workup to the individual needs of the patient.

Take-Home Points

- When lab tests are ordered during the workup of erectile dysfunction, it is important to know what the physician is looking for prior to having a test.
- Ordering every test on every patient is not necessary. If a physician orders every test without an explanation, find another physician.
- Prior to proceeding with venous leakage surgery, it

is important that you have an adequate diagnosis. This necessitates a minimal workup: a Duplex Doppler ultrasound examination and a cavernosogram.

- Rigiscan testing is not for all patients with erectile dysfunction, but if there is any question as to cause, it is a useful test.

- Prior to having a rigiscan, be sure that your insurance carrier recognizes this as a covered service.

- Before proceeding with a surgical procedure on the penis, it is recommended to have a rigiscan to document poor erectile functioning, especially prior to a penile implant.

- Only candidates for microvascular reconstructive surgery should undergo arteriography.

- Microvascular reconstructive surgery should be limited to very experienced surgeons.

Chapter 5

Priapism, Ejaculatory Disorders, and Peyronie's Disease

Priapism

Priapism is the occurrence of any persistent erection for more than four hours duration in the absence of sexual stimulation. Priapism is named after Priapus, the Greek god of fertility, and the son of Aphrodite, the goddess of love. He was apparently an ugly, satyrlike man with enormous genitalia. He was the god of gardens, bees, goats, and sheep. According to the story, Priapus had a huge tongue, a fat belly, and his penis was so large that he was restricted to the position of scarecrow in the fields.

Most erections due to sexual stimulation never approach four to six hours. Priapism is not associated with sexual excitement, at least not initially, and the erection does not subside after ejaculation. Priapism can occur in all age groups, including newborns. Most cases of priapism are clustered between two age groups: between the ages of five to ten and twenty to fifty years. Priapism constitutes a true urologic emergency. Men often joke that they wish they could have a permanent erection, but in reality, men are extremely miserable when this actually happens.

Many physicians have characterized priapism in different ways. I find it simplest to classify it by what caused it. Children with priapism are typically those who have leukemia. In this situation, the white blood cells occlude, or block the outflow of blood from the penis causing priapism. Also, children with sickle-cell disease can be afflicted with priapism. In this situation, the penis receives low oxygen, and therefore, the blood sickles and prevents outflow because of sludging. Other rare causes of priapism in childhood include trauma, either to the penis or to the area underneath the penis known as the *perineum*. Additionally, spinal cord injuries can cause priapism. Extremely rare causes of priapism include drug side effects, but typically these drugs are not used in children.

In adults, priapism either has a known cause or an unknown cause, in which case it is idiopathic, or has no identifiable cause. Typical causes in adults include sickle-cell disease, which accounts for almost a third of all cases. It is reported that 42 percent of all sickle-cell adults and 64 percent of all sickle-cell children will eventually develop priapism.

The most common cause of priapism is pharmacological injection therapy, which far outshadows all currently known causes. Drug-related priapism includes those drugs used to treat psychotic type illnesses, including thorazine and chlorpromazine. Other more uncommon drugs include those used to treat high-blood pressure such as prazosin. Rare causes may also be related to cancers that can infiltrate the penis and prevent the outflow of blood.

Once a diagnosis is made, it is extremely important to get prompt treatment. The diagnosis is not difficult. It is a painful erection unrelated to sexual stimulation. One of the key factors in the examination is that the glans is not tumescent, or swollen.

The length of time the erection has been present should be carefully documented. It is also important to document what medications the patient has been taking, including any use of illicit drugs such as marijuana, which has also been linked to priapism. It is also important to get an idea of how long the erections normally last and if there has been associated trauma. Following a medical history, a careful physical examination should reveal a hard penis with a soft glans. It is also important to check the rectum and the abdomen for evidence of unusual cancers and the other causes of priapism. The goal of all treatment modalities is to make the erection go away and preserve future erectile functioning. The faster we can get the erection to subside, the better the outcome.

Once priapism and its source have been identified, it is categorized into two major types: low-flow priapism or ischemic, which means that little or no blood flow is getting to the penis and this lack can cause damage; or high-flow priapism, which is the result of trauma to the penis. In this case, there is actually a large amount of blood flow to the penis. Our first step after the careful history and physical examination is to obtain a blood-gas measurement of the blood from the penis. This provides a clue as to how long the condition has been present and how much damage has occurred. A small needle is placed in the penis; some of the blood is aspirated and then sent to a lab for determination. This will also help categorize whether the cause of the priapism is low flow or high flow.

If a patient gets treatment within four to six hours, the erection can almost always be reduced with medication. My first step for the patient with priapism of less than four hours duration is the use of decongestant medications. These medications include drugs such as pseudoephedrine and terbutaline, which may act to decrease blood flow to the penis and is very successful in early cases. If the erection does not respond, I then proceed with aspiration. The longer the condition goes without treatment, the worse the prognosis. Once the blood-gas measurement has been performed and the priapism is determined to be ischemic, or that in fact the penis has very poor blood flow, I then evacuate the old blood by aspirating through a small needle placed directly in the corporal body. This is done by first cleansing the area, then infiltrating the local anesthetic over the skin of the penis and placing the needle. I withdraw 50 to 150 ccs of old blood. This allows the penis to detumesce.

If treatment is done early in the course of the disease, this is all that is necessary. However, if the erection begins to recur, certain vaso-active type drugs including epinephrine may be instilled, causing the blood vessels to constrict and prevent priapism from recurring.

If this is unsuccessful, a shunting procedure is performed. This is a minor surgical procedure that can be done in the

H.A. was a medical professional who had read about the treatment of erectile dysfunction with penile injections. He injected himself with a dose that far exceeded what he needed. He developed a rock-hard penis and enjoyed it for several hours. Unfortunately, he developed priapism. He was so embarrassed by this that he actually went for seven days before seeking medical help. The pain was excruciating, and he tried numerous treatments that he had read about in outdated medical journals including ice water enemas and injecting local anesthetic into the penis. The resulting erection was unsalvageable, and the patient was eventually left with a penis that was less than an inch long. The caveat to this scenario is early treatment for priapism is essential to prevent permanent loss of the penis.

emergency room. It allows the blood to drain from the corporal body into the glans and surrounding tissues. Numerous shunts are named after the people who have performed these surgeries. As you can imagine, the more names and procedures associated with a medical condition means that there is no perfect answer. We generally do the best job we can to prevent recurrence.

Timing is the most important issue with priapism. Treatment must be performed on the ischemic priapism as soon as possible to prevent permanent damage. Tight dressings after the procedure may also result in damage to the skin and loss of tissue. It is extremely important to have the physician get an informed consent and to be absolutely sure that the patient understands that at least 50 percent of men who develop priapism will have some degree of erection problems, regardless of the duration or method of management used to treat this condition.

Complications can and do occur during and after the treatment for priapism. These complications include:

- recurrence of priapism
- bleeding from the holes placed in the penis as a part of the shunting procedure
- infections
- skin necrosis
- infection of the corporal body
- infection of the skin around it
- damage to the urethra and the urine tube, including strictures
- holes between the urethra and the skin
- loss of the penis

Loss of the penis is a situation that does happen, and I have personally seen and been involved with it. Infection is so common that all patients with priapism should be placed on antibiotics. In rare cases, people may have a blood clot form in the penis after shunting procedures that can break off and go to the heart causing death from a condition called a *pulmonary embolus*.

The best way to avoid priapism is to be alert when it happens. When it occurs, go to an emergency room where there is a urologist present. If you are using penile injections and the erection lasts more than two or three hours, I recommend taking a pseudoephedrine, over-the-counter decongestant that successfully abates many cases of poten-

M.F. was a farmer who was struck in the perineum while working with a power take-off instrument. He developed a traumatic high-flow priapism because an artery had ruptured; the blood entered the artery, went into the corporal body, and created an erection, then immediately left it because the veins were not constricted. Careful history, physical examination, and determination of the blood gases made the diagnosis. Finally an arteriogram of the pudendal arterial system was done, and this identified the point of the fistula. A small coil of material was placed into the damaged artery and prevented the erection. The patient eventually recovered and is currently able to get normal erections. The caveat in this case is that it is extremely important to have an actual accurate diagnosis when treating this disease. Irrigations with drugs and shunts would have been hopeless in this situation and would have made the patient worse off.

tial priapism. Most non-urologists have little if any experience in treating priapism. A high index suspicion, a careful history and physical, and a careful, specialized treatment plan are essential in the successful management of priapism.

Ejaculatory Disorders

Most of my discussions with patients about ejaculation centers around education. Many individuals confuse an orgasm with an ejaculation. The two are extremely different.

Generally, an ejaculation is a reflex event of a highly limited length of time and represents numerous levels of neural input.

Ejaculations from a nervous system standpoint can happen in two ways. The first is purely a central nervous system standpoint, as with a young man who has a nocturnal emission, or a wet dream. This is a combination of erotic stimulation during sleep combined with some limited amount of friction. The majority of contribution is from the central nervous system and results in an ejaculation. This generally occurs in younger patients and oftentimes in an older man who, for a variety of reasons, is not having active intercourse or ejaculating on a regular basis.

The impulse goes into the spinal cord and then into the brain where the automatic nervous system stimulates the sympathetic portion of the autonomic nervous system, which results in a contraction of the male accessory sexual organs including the vas deferens, the prostate, and the bladder neck. This is a fancy way to say that the brain stimulates the sympathetic nervous system into creating the ejaculate to be squeezed and expelled. This process is a seminal emission, in which the semen, the fluid from both the prostate fluid and the seminal vesicles, is deposited into the back part of the urethra.

An ejaculation occurs when this fluid is propelled out of the penis. This occurs when there is a contraction of the bulbocavernosus muscles, or more commonly referred to as an orgasm. An orgasm is the actual contraction of these muscles expelling the fluid. It is possible to have an orgasm without the expelling of fluid. It is also possible to have the fluid go backward into the bladder, which is called a *retro-*

grade ejaculation. This is most commonly seen in men who have had prostate surgery or men who have had surgery to damage the sympathetic nerves.

Additionally, some men will have a failure of emission. In other words, the fluid will not be deposited, and therefore, the ejaculate is dry. A typical ejaculate is between 2 and 5 ccs, or roughly one tablespoon.

There is a great deal of ignorance about exactly what an ejaculation is and what can cause it. Ejaculatory disorders have numerous causes. The most common ejaculatory diagnosis is premature ejaculation. Many times, simply discussing premature ejaculation and the physiology associated with it convinces the patient that it is not a problem to worry about. I always use the analogy of our ancient predecessors: Early man would not have evolved had he not been a premature ejaculator. In other words, if reproduction took long periods of penile-vaginal penetration before an ejaculation occurred, humankind would not have evolved. It is much more important from a survival standpoint to have a quick ejaculation with multiple partners for preservation of our species.

Also, partner education is important to explain the importance of timing and the frequency of sexual intercourse. I always try to educate at this juncture since so many men have learned their ejaculatory physiology from pornographic movies in which it is common to see men with sustained erections for long periods of time and ejaculations that appear to constitute a gallon of fluid.

Neurologic lesions at any level can also cause ejaculatory dysfunction. Men with spinal cord lesions caused by an injury or surgical damage can have an inability to ejaculate, such as in men who have had colon surgery or abdominal aortic surgery. Because the sympathetic nerves lie so close to the structures that control sexual functioning, they can easily be damaged at the time of surgery.

Other problems, such as diabetes and multiple sclerosis, are other causes of ejaculatory problems. Many drugs can cause a lack of emission, which is a failure of deposition of the seminal fluid into the posterior or back part of the urethra, and result in a failure of ejaculation. Hypertensives and cold medications potentially fall into this category. Damage to the structures that propel the fluid from the penis outward, such as bladder neck damage, is also a cause of ejaculatory disorders. The most common form of this is in men who have had prostate surgery, particularly a transurethral resection of the prostate (TURP) where the bladder neck is destroyed and the resulting condition is retrograde ejaculation. Perhaps the most common form of ejaculatory dysfunction is premature ejaculation. But an accurate diagnosis requires a satisfactory definition.

The definition of premature ejaculation varies for every individual and depends on the person. I have seen many persons who are able to sustain intercourse for five and ten minutes and yet complain of premature ejaculation. I've also seen many men who ejaculate before even penetrating the vagina. Other ejaculatory dysfunction problems, although less common, are men who can sustain erection and are able to penetrate for long periods of time but often do not ejaculate. This may sound like a wonderful thing, but in fact it is not.

The most troubling situation for men is a bloody ejaculation. This is usually a benign, self-limited condition called

Y.M. was brought to the clinic by his wife for evaluation. She said he was a premature ejaculator, and it was impossible to have relations with him because of this problem. A careful history revealed that he ejaculated even before he was able to penetrate, and when he did his wife became so angry that there would be a long period before he would be allowed to attempt intercourse again. Creating this atmosphere of hostility greatly exacerbated his problem. The use of serotonin uptake inhibitors provided dramatic results in this situation.

hematospermia. It typically relates either to inflammation of the seminal vesicles (the structure that stores fluid prior to ejaculation), the colon, or the prostate. Observation and antibiotics will easily treat this condition, and it is rarely associated with a malignancy. A careful examination by a doctor can easily rule out this possibility. The most appropriate measure is that of reassurance. Then it typically ceases to be much of a problem.

When I examine men who have had an ejaculatory dysfunction, I take a careful history focusing on the frequency of sexual intercourse. Infrequent intercourse is the most common cause of premature ejaculation. I also focus on changes in sexual functioning, particularly about the time of ejaculation, and on things such as painful ejaculation, blood in the ejaculate, decreased ejaculate volume, and sudden decreases in the volume of the ejaculate versus a chronically low ejaculatory volume. Again, the physical examination is important to carefully examine the prostate and collecting structures.

The treatment of ejaculatory disorders has undergone a renaissance. We are now able to effectively treat most problems with targeted medications, depending upon the diagnosis. Before the advent of these medications, mental health individuals and sexual therapists saw most of these patients. Premature ejaculation was commonly believed to be a psychological problem. Treatment involved only behavioral therapy, which required intense motivation from both partners and which typically did not achieve the success rate as reported in the standard literature of the time. This therapy involved sexual foreplay to the point of ejaculation, without allowing ejaculation to occur, then slowly increasing the length of time between activity and the point of ejaculation.

Previous medical therapy used local anesthetics, a non-prescriptive cream found in drugstores. Men would apply roughly one-half teaspoon of this anesthetic jelly to the penis and wear a condom. Approximately thirty minutes later, sexual relations were initiated. Treatment could be successful, but an obvious side effect was vaginal anesthesia. Before the advent of serotonin uptake blockers, another treatment involved giving the patient penile injections to create an erection that would not go away after premature ejaculation, thus allowing the individual to get over the fear of premature ejaculation.

The advent of serotonin uptake blockers has changed the treatment of ejaculatory disorders dramatically. It has been found that men who are on selective serotonin reuptake inhibitors (SSRIs) to treat depression have difficulty ejaculating, and many patients complained about this side effect. This observation led many physicians to use this side effect

J.F. had substantial problems sustaining intercourse. Apparently, his wife told him (at that time) that
they were allowed to have intercourse at a rigidly set
period of time. If he was unable to sustain an erection for a period that would provide her with satisfaction, she would then terminate the event. This
created an intense problem for the partner, and he was
basically unable to perform and became a premature
ejaculator. This problem was resolved when he termi-
nated the relationship.

as a treatment in men with premature ejaculation. These
medications, including fluoxetine and sertraline, prolong
ejaculatory latency and increase the time it takes to ejaculate by up to thirty minutes.

It is extremely important to note that these drugs are not
currently indicated for this treatment, and their usage must
be done with caution and only by informed individuals since
this is an off-label use of these medications. I recommend
using the lower-strength dosage roughly four hours prior to
anticipated sexual relations. I have found it to have a high
success rate.

Peyronie's Disease

Peyronie's disease was described in 1743 by a French
physician named François de la Peyroni, who reported that
patients with scar tissue in the penis had a significantly
bent penis. Until recently, Peyronie's disease was a poorly

understood condition. Many original descriptions depicted it as secondary to scarring from masturbation or sexually transmitted diseases. It is not a malignant condition of the penis. It affects men primarily between the ages of forty to sixty. The reported incidence is somewhere in the range of 4 percent, but I suspect it is much more common and vastly underreported. Patients often delay seeking medical help out of fear and embarrassment. The hallmark of the disease is a plaque or hard spot along the shaft of the penis. This occurs in the vast majority of men with Peyronie's disease. The plaque may range from a few millimeters or may encompass the entire length of the penis. The most common reason for seeking medical help is painful erections and erectile dysfunction.

The cause of Peyronie's disease is not well understood. Currently, a number of theories implicate trauma as the most likely cause. In the cases that I have seen in my practice, this is the most common cause. Unfortunately, as with most things that relate to human sexuality, we are not taught how to have intercourse. Consequently, many positions and practices that young men do put a great deal of torque and pressure on the penis, causing microtrauma to its delicate supportive structures.

When there is microdamage, scar tissue develops and restricts the blood flow to the area. It either impedes the blood flow, causing erectile dysfunction, or it causes a bending in the penis at the level of the scar. Occasionally, this bend is so severe that is makes intercourse impossible.

Peyronie's disease has also been linked to family history. Although this is a difficult linkage, since many men don't really know if their family had a history of it, enough reports support this as a risk factor. Peyronie's disease has even been implicated with certain medications such as beta-blockers, the medications used in the treatment of high blood pressure. Other fibrosing-type diseases such as Dupuytren's contracture, a disease that causes visible scarring of the palms and soles, have also been linked to Peyronie's disease.

The natural history of Peyronie's disease is variable. The disease has an acute and a chronic phase. The acute phase is variable, but the majority of the scarring and the bending occur during this phase. The chronic phase may last for long periods of time. Typically, roughly 50 percent of patients with Peyronie's disease will improve with time, and 50 percent will get worse with time. One study found that almost half the patients never experienced the problems with bending of the penis, and typically, the pain associated with the acute phase of the disease resolved with time.

There have been numerous attempts at both medical and surgical treatments for this disease. Medical management has encompassed everything under the sun, but because there is no clear reason for the disease, there is no clear treatment for it. People have advocated the use of spa waters, mercury, arsenic, radiation treatments, ultrasound treatments, shortwave laser treatments, and shock wave treatments for this condition. None of these have found wide acceptance because none have been proven to be effective.

The only real oral treatment that has been widely available is vitamin E because of its antioxidant properties and Potaba (potassium amino benzoate). The Food and Drug Administration has classified it as a "possibly effective drug," although the mechanism of action is not well understood.

Numerous studies have examined the use of other drugs.

These include tamoxifen, an anti-estrogen drug used in the treatment of breast cancer. There is no long-term data available on the use of this drug.

Finally, a recent study advocated the use of oral colchicine, an anti-inflammatory drug used in the treatment of acute gout which inhibits the motion of white blood cells and prevents pain in the acute phase of arthritis. This is a complex medication and has been used to treat numerous conditions. Side effects include diarrhea, and it has been associated with erectile dysfunction as well. For years people have used intralesional steroids where they have actually injected long-acting steroids into the plaque of the penis to prevent the fibrosis from occurring. Again, there is no long-term data available with regard to this procedure.

Unfortunately, at this time there is no definitive treatment for Peyronie's disease. In my own clinical practice, I tend to shy away from Potaba as a first-line therapy because of the large doses required and the side effects. People complain of gastrointestinal distress as well as the cost of the medication. I recommend vitamin E as the first-line medical therapy because it has been shown to have other benefits in the body, and it is not harmful in the recommended doses. There is, however, no control study that demonstrates its benefit.

Surgical Treatment

The surgical treatment of Peyronie's disease is similar to the medical treatment—there is no best operation. Before considering a surgical procedure, the disease should be stable for one year. This avoids surgery on the man who may get a spontaneous resolution of the disease. Surgery should only be performed on men who have difficulty inserting the penis during intercourse because of angulation. If a patient has somewhat of a bend but is able to enjoy intercourse, I do not recommend surgery. As long as the penis can remain firm enough for penetration and relatively straight enough for intercourse, I do not recommend therapy other than the use of vitamin E.

Surgeons visualize the degree of bending prior to surgery by taking Polaroid pictures of both the side and top view. The most important question is, "How firm is the penis past the narrowing or the scar?" This will determine if, in addition to the straightening procedure, something else needs to be done. The Nesbit procedure is the gold standard procedure for the treatment of Peyronie's disease. This procedure was developed to taper the unaffected corporal body on the side to correct the deformity. In other words, with a substantial bend, we take segments from the corporal body on the opposite side to create a straight penis.

As with all operations, the Nesbit procedure has numerous complications which must be carefully discussed with the prospective patient. They can include postoperative difficulty with erections, over-correcting or bending to the opposite side, scarring, numbness of the glans or the penile shaft, blood collection under the skin of the penis called a *hematoma*, and wound infection. It is important to advise patients that this operation will not remove plaque. Tissues are merely shifted around to accommodate for the scarring the plaque has caused.

Other modified procedures use a plication technique. Instead of cutting wedges into the corporal body, as with the

Nesbit procedure, a plication pulls the tissues together by putting multiple loops of sutures farther away from each other. This actually accomplishes what the Nesbit procedure does but on a less traumatic scale. It is a much less invasive technique, and the results are similar. In addition to using modified procedures for Peyronie's disease, the plication technique is also useful treating congenital curvature of the penis, a relatively uncommon condition in young men. It is also possible to excise plaques and use grafts of artificial material such as Gore-Tex or the patient's skin without its outer lining. Gore-Tex is a product commonly found in waterproof clothing and has been successful in arterial grafts. It was originally developed as a coating for wire, but it has found a multitude of other uses, including grafts.

Penile prosthesis is another surgical procedure to repair this condition. Prosthesis not only straightens the penis but improves the erection. A careful history and physical examination should first establish that this is in fact a stable disease, and then to maximize medical therapy which includes vitamin E. Men who are unable to have intercourse because of a significant bend but still have a hard penis can get penile injections at the office to observe firsthand how hard the erection is as well as any other complications.

Additionally, I recommend a rigiscan to compare the base to the tip. If the penis is severely bent but the erection is firm, I recommend only a straightening procedure. Graft material is not the initial treatment in my practice. If the penis is so severely bent that the tip is soft, surgically straightening the penis will still require an additional method to improve erections, such as a vacuum erection device or penile injections. At this juncture, I recommend a penile implant in men who do not wish to have additional treatments.

A penile prosthesis will straighten the curvature without the need for incision of the plaque. Additionally, patients will not need some type of grafting procedure with the prosthesis. Placement of a prosthesis in men with Peyronie's disease is no more difficult than with most other patients. But I feel that Peyronie's patients with a substantial bend that precludes adequate penetration and who are impotent are the only candidates for prosthesis. There is no perfect surgical treatment for this condition, which is why there are so many treatment options. My recommendations to patients are: Be comfortable with the diagnosis to at least face the treatment initially; and before considering surgical therapy, be sure that the physician you have chosen is experienced in this type of surgery.

Unusual Problems

Some of the more unusual scenarios I see in a urologic practice that focuses on sexual dysfunction are quite uncommon, but they can have some bearing on male sexual dysfunction.

Penile Fracture

Fractures to the penis, although uncommon, do occur. Discussing this in casual terms almost always causes men to cross their legs in response to the mere thought of this catastrophe. Even seasoned medical professionals cringe. Many physicians don't understand the underlying mechanism of this injury.

V.E. was a twenty-nine-year-old man who was urinating with a morning erection. His penis got caught between the seat and the rim of the toilet. Upon standing up, he snapped his penis, and caused a disruption of the right shaft of the corporal body.

Penile fracture can only occur with an erection. The vast majority of these injuries occur with sexual activity, although I have personally seen cases of a fractured penis that resulted when a man rolled on top of an erect penis while sleeping.

Penile fractures can also happen during masturbation. In one case, a teenager who was masturbating forced his erect penis into his jeans at the fear of discovery and fractured it. The vast majority of patients are so embarrassed they will often manufacture elaborate stories. In these scenarios, the old adage "truth is stranger than fiction" becomes significant. I have never seen a penile fracture in a man with a short penis. Fractures typically occur in men with longer-than-average penises, although I am certain it can happen in the whole spectrum of penis sizes. The symptom complex is fairly classic. Typically the partner is on top, the penis becomes dislodged from the vagina and in an attempt to reinsert it, the partner will come down on the penis, striking the symphysis pubis, the female pelvic bone, just missing the vaginal opening, and creating a sudden bending. A loud snap and excruciating pain always follows, as well as the rapid development of a hematoma or bruise. Roughly 20 percent of the men will have an associated urethral injury as well. These injuries are not difficult to diagnose, and symptoms will depend upon the severity of the fracture.

Men with penile fractures are in excruciating pain and have a black-and-blue penis. When the diagnosis is equivocal—that is, there is a large bruise, but no obvious distortion or destruction—the penis is evaluated with corporal cavernosography. The urologist or radiologist places a fine needle into the corporal body of the penis and injects contrast material in order to examine the shape of the corporal bodies and to look for leakage. If there is a question of urethral injury, a retrograde urethrogram is also performed in which contrast material is instilled down the urethra via a small tube or catheter to look for leakage. Urethral injury is usually evident with blood in the urine at the time of the workup.

Surgery is the best treatment for fractures. The faster the torn tissues can be reapproximated, the better the healing process. The problem with conservative management is that fibrosis of the lining of the corporal body can create a bend and poor healing, as with a broken arm. Additionally, complications from expanding blood clots, such as a blood clot accumulation or a hematoma, or an infection of the hematoma can occur. These men with penile fractures are typically young, sexually active, and highly motivated to resume sexual activity as soon as the healing process is complete so surgery is often the best treatment.

Blunt Injuries

Blunt injuries are the result of a crush injury to the penis, such as something striking an erection. I have seen a case in which a man caught his erect penis in a door. In another case, a drug dealer angered a supplier, and his punishment was to place his penis on the ground and have it stomped

B.F. was a thirty-four-year-old man who was having intercourse with his girlfriend in the superior position. His penis became dislodged when his partner moved in an upward fashion. Not realizing that it had slipped out, she came down with all of her weight and snapped his penis in two. This affected both corporal bodies as well as the urethra. This case underscores the need to take care in certain sexual positions so as not to submit the penis to excessive forces.

on with the man's heel, thereby crushing the corporal bodies and the urethra. This painful event needed immediate surgical attention.

Penile Trauma

Some of the more unusual cases include loss of the penile skin. Because the skin of the penis is so loose and mobile it is easily caught in power devices or zippers. Foreskin may get caught in a zipper, requiring excision of the area. This is usually more frightening than painful.

Foreign Objects

Foreign objects found in the urethra and rectum relate to aberrant sexual practices. In some cases, devices or even pencils are inserted into the urethra while masturbating around it. The danger in this situation is damage to the urethra and potential loss of the object if it happens to migrate back into the bladder. In Asian cultures it is popular for men to have plastic or silicone beads implanted under the skin of the penis to increase sexual pleasure for the female partner. This can sometimes become infected. Some men have had a constricting band become lodged at the base of the penis. Although these constriction bands are not a common sexual practice, they are widely available. We recommend that constriction bands be used only with vacuum erection devices or after a diagnosis of venous leak.

Take-Home Points

- Priapism is a urologic emergency. Treatment of priapism should be done by an experienced physician. This is typically a urologist.

- When using pharmocologic injection therapy, use of over-the-counter decongestants can frequently abate a priaptic episode, and I encourage their use when an erection lasts more than two or three hours.

- The definition of premature ejaculation is arbitrary. It is different for all men, and depends upon the sexual partner.

- The secret to avoiding premature ejaculation is increasing the frequency of sexual intercourse.

- It is important to ejaculate on a regular basis.

- Avoid sexual positions that put undue strain on your penis.

- Always opt for the least invasive treatment before proceeding to a surgical treatment.

- If considering an exotic surgical procedure such as a Gore-Tex graft to the penis, think about an implant before proceeding in this fashion, and go to a urologist who has a significant amount of experience in these types of procedures.

Chapter 6

Testosterone Replacement Therapy

Androgens

The use of testosterone is widespread. Previous reported uses include infertility, athletic enhancement, erectile dysfunction and libido problems. Their use can have grave consequences if not used prudently. Androgen, or more specifically testosterone, is widely utilized to treat erectile dysfunction. The classic theory about testosterone treatment is that it stimulates the sex drive and, by doing so, restores erectile functioning.

True androgen deficiency is an uncommon diagnosis. Individuals with truly low androgen levels have dramatically augmented their sex drives with the use of testosterone. Because testosterone affects the skin, bone, and skeletal muscle, as well as blood lipids and blood cells, these men generally have muscle weakness, muscle atrophy, little facial and body hair, and a female escutcheon. Depending on what age the deficiency occurred, there may also be changes in the size of the genitalia.

Following a careful history and physical examination, the only accurate way to diagnose the low testosterone state is by measuring the serum level of testosterone. This is a simple blood test that any commercial laboratory can do. At different points during the day, testosterone levels may be widely variable. The human body is cyclical. For example, our state of restfulness or wakefulness varies at different times of the day just as testosterone levels vary.

Serum testing measures testosterone levels in the body. Initially, the hormone that exists in the serum may be bound to a protein that allows it to be transported in the body. This protein is called sex hormone binding globulin (SHBG). The total testosterone consists of two forms of testosterone; one is bound to SHBG and the other is free circulating testosterone unattached to serum proteins. In conditions such as hypothyroidism and cirrhosis, measurement of the total testosterone level may be normal but the patient may have symptoms of low testosterone. In these conditions, the SHBG is increased and this decreases the amount of testosterone that is available for use. The opposite is true where SHBG is decreased and the free testosterone levels are high. This situation is seen in men with obesity and hypothyroidism. These men have normal amounts of testosterone available for use by the body but the serum testosterone level is decreased. Generally, your physician will make the determination of whether to obtain a test measure for both total and free testosterone levels. I usually reserve this in clinical situations where I am suspicious.

Once it has been determined that the testosterone level is low, measuring the luteinizing hormone (LH) can help determine the cause. This separates the patients who have testicular disease from those who have diseases of the pituitary gland, the master gland that sits at the base of the brain and essentially controls many bodily functions. A low testosterone level may indicate an elevated prolactin level as well, a condition known as a *hyperprolactinoma*. Elevated prolactin can decrease testosterone levels by decreasing the secretion of the hormone that tells the testicle to produce testosterone.

Several things must be weighed before beginning testosterone replacement therapy. In most clinical practice, men are simply given a course of testosterone injections over several months to see if it improves the erectile functioning. This is common in a primary care setting but unfortunately it rarely produces improvement.

Some causes of low testosterone levels include congenital problems (such as deficiencies of male hormones and rare malformation syndromes), and acquired problems, including aging, chronic illness, drugs, starvation, stress, head trauma, infections, cancers, surgeries, alcoholism, removal of or trauma to the testicles, and infection or twisting of the testicles in their sack. This is just a small portion of a long list of possible causes. Another factor is whether or not the testosterone is bound by SHBG. High-fat diets, for example, affect SHBG. Also, certain drugs compete with testosterone in the body, such as spironolactone, an antihypertensive, and danazol, a drug used to treat certain breast conditions in women.

R.Y. was a fifty-one-year-old man who had lethargy and erectile dysfunction. Upon examination he was found to have a normal phallus but very small, firm testicles. He had sparse facial hair and indicated that he shaved only once every week, if even that often. His serum testosterone level was less than 100. His diagnosis was mumps orchitis. He had contracted mumps when he was nineteen, and it had affected both testicles. He was started on testos-terone supplementation at a dose of 200 mg every three weeks, which his wife administered. The results were dramatic. He gained weight, began shaving daily, and was able to have sustained intercourse on a regular basis.

Men with low testosterone levels can improve their libido with testosterone treatment. Once a man is diagnosed as hypogonadic, or having a low testosterone level, the next step is to choose which form of treatment to utilize. As with all medications, benefits must be weighed against the numer-ous risks. Age is one important factor in making this deci-sion. In men less than fifty years old, the goal is to restore libido and erections. Some of the side benefits include preser-vation of bone mass, much in the same way estrogen helps prevent osteoporosis in menopausal women. Testosterone also improves strength, physical stamina, and general well-being. It almost sounds like this is the perfect drug.

The downside of testosterone is that it can increase serum cholesterol. It can also increase the growth of the prostate, and if early-stage prostate cancer is present, treatment may stimulate wild growth. The analogy I use with patients is that testosterone treatment is like throwing Miracle Grow on a patch of weeds. So it is extremely important to be sure you don't have prostate cancer before beginning testosterone replacement therapy.

Testosterone preparations are as numerous as the causes for low testosterone. Physicians have a host of choices, including oral or sublingual preparations, patches, pellets, and shots. In the injectable category there are numerous short-acting and long-acting preparations. We will briefly discuss each of the preparations and the risks and benefits of each.

Before beginning testosterone replacement therapy, I also recommend monitoring prostate-specific antigen (PSA) levels. The PSA is a useful marker that aids in the diagnosis and management of prostate cancer. It is extremely important to know the baseline PSA before beginning therapy. I also check baseline liver function to be sure that there is no liver damage prior to testosterone therapy, and finally, I do a baseline blood lipid test. I then monitor the blood lipids at least twice a year. I carefully counsel the patient about the potential downfall of this type of therapy since long-term testosterone therapy has been associated with prostate cancer. Men who have low levels of testosterone are still at risk for prostate cancer.

Oral Preparations

The major drawback to oral preparations of testosterone is the fact that they must be in a form that will allow their absorption from the GI tract. In other words, they are taken by mouth as an inactive form, absorbed, and then activated in the liver, a process known as *methylation*. Unfortunately, this is not an ideal situation as these preparations are fraught with liver dysfunction. Additionally, the half-life of these preparations is very short, and they must be taken throughout the day.

The oral preparations available in the United States are perhaps the least desirable way to replace testosterone, and I personally feel that there are no indications to use these in replacement therapy. Other oral preparations available outside the United States are reported to be somewhat better. They are compounded with medications that allow the testosterone to bypass the liver and avoid liver toxicity. Unfortunately, these are not currently available in the United States.

Transdermal Preparations

Two transdermal preparations are widely available. The first and original is a patch worn on the scrotum. The scrotal skin is ideal, not because of its position but because of its unique properties that allow the testosterone to absorb into the skin. The scrotal skin is thinner and has a higher circulation than other skin surfaces. This type of treatment has a low incidence of side effects, but the major drawback is the need to shave the scrotum on a fairly regular basis and to use a hairdryer to apply it. This preparation, unfortunately, has not become extremely popular.

Recently, another testosterone replacement preparation has been approved that uses the unique delivery system of daily placing the patch on the torso. With this method, serum testosterone levels remain stable, unlike the wide swings of the injection method, and patients can thereby avoid the monthly injections. Downsides, however, include skin lesions and dermatitis, and it is expensive. Common skin rashes can be avoided by pretreatment with cortisone creams. Also, many patients who prefer the transdermal route have third party insurance plans that pay for prescription medications because the cost is prohibitive for men who are on chronic replacement therapy.

Both preparations are widely available, and it is certainly important to discuss these options with your physician when considering testosterone replacement therapy.

Injections

Currently, the most popular method of testosterone supplementation is by injection. The most common compound and the ones used for decades in the United States are testosterone cypionate and testosterone enanthate. These are generally given as a 200-mg injection every two to three weeks. Results are usually satisfactory for the majority of patients.

The downside to this has been an initial super-physiologic testosterone level during the first few days after the injection followed by a decrease. In other words, when you first get the injection, the testosterone level goes much higher than natural levels would be, and then tends to drop. This creates a peak-and-valley situation. It is usually not noticeable to patients. Some physicians, however, feel that the intermittent elevations may have more long-term consequences than a steady level produced by transdermal preparations.

Studies are currently investigating whether transdermal

R.B. was a fifty-one-year-old executive. He had a
sudden loss of interest in sexual relations. A careful
history revealed that he was able to achieve an erection but had no desire in having intercourse. He had
recently remarried, and the relationship had initially
been extremely physical. His testosterone level was
extremely low, and further evaluation indicated a high
serum prolactin level. He indicated that he also had
double vision and headaches as well. His diagnosis
was a prolactinoma; a small prolactin-secreting
tumor at the base of the brain in the area known as the
pituitary. Treatment with the drug bromocriptine was
dramatic and has totally resolved the problem.

testosterone has advantages over testosterone shots. Again,
this is not a clear situation, and so it is important to discuss
this with your physician. In my clinical practice, most
patients choose testosterone injections because of cost consid-
erations. I generally teach patients or their partners how to
give the injection, and then prescribe the appropriate dosages.
Cost is roughly $10 for a 10-cc vial, which is good for up
to fifteen weeks. It is the most cost-effective option available.

Other types of testosterone preparations include testosterone pellets that can be implanted much the same as the
Norplant, although this is not available worldwide. Studies
are also looking at testosterone given under the tongue, or
sublingually. The most important take-home message in this
situation is that each testosterone delivery system has its
benefits and side effects. It is important that both patient
and physician understand them thoroughly.

The current recommendation for men about to undergo testosterone replacement therapy is either the transdermal or transcrotal patch or testosterone cypionate injections, 200 mg every two weeks, or 400 mg every month. The downside to the 400 mg dose is that the peak-and-valley effect is more dramatic than with the 200-mg treatments. Men on 400 mg should be carefully watched for signs of liver toxicity as well as changes in the blood lipids.

Herbal Treatments

The most important message about using herbal treatments for any medical condition is that herbs are strong medications. The only difference between herbs and drugs is that the drugs have gone through extensive randomized testing while herbs have not. Many herbs have powerful effects on genital tissues, and erectile dysfunction is no different than any other type of medical problem. I'll review some of the more common herbs known to help sexual potency and those that may cause erectile dysfunction.

Table 6.1   Common Herbal Treatments

Damiana:	Damiana is reported to improve blood flow to genital areas. This herb stimulates muscle contractions in the intestinal tract and apparently improves blood flow to the genital tract. It has been used as a sexuality tonic for women as well. It is of unknown benefit.

continued

Table 6.1   *Continued*

Sarsaparilla: This has been reputed to be a male
                hormonelike substance for men that can
                improve libido. It is of unknown benefit.

Pygeum: The extract of African prunes has been
                reported to be beneficial in men with
                prostrate problems. It is commonly
                included in many herbal preparations. Its
                effectiveness in men with erectile
                dysfunction is unknown.

Saw   Saw palmetto berries contain a five alpha
palmetto   reductase inhibitor and is very similar to
berry: the drug currently marketed to shrink the
                prostate. Men should take great caution
                with this medication because it will also
                decrease the ejaculate volume when taken
                for long periods of time. It is very effective
                in men with prostate problems and is
                widely utilized.

Ginkgo   This extract has been shown in numerous
biloba: studies to increase blood flow in the body.
                Some studies show that it is as good as
                other medications used to treat senility
                disorders. It has been recommended to
                improve blood flow to the male genitals.
                This claim is as yet unsubstantiated.

Table 6.1   *Continued*

DHEA:	Dehydroepiandrosterone (DHEA) is a naturally occurring hormone in the body. It has no known role. Its levels are high at puberty and slowly drop off with age. It was originally banned in 1985 but has now reoccurred as a dietary supplement that does not require FDA approval. There are no proven benefits to DHEA supplements, but there are significant risks. Large doses can aggravate prostate problems and may even be linked to early prostate cancer. This, of course, is totally unproven at this point, but I recommend taking it with great caution.
Ephedra:	Ephedra, which contains the drug ephedrine, has been used for bronchial asthma and acts as the precursor to many of the drugs that help stimulate the central nervous system. Major side effects of this drug are difficulty achieving an erection, and difficulty ejaculating. This drug has also been linked to high blood pressure, and many deaths have been linked to this as a consequence of strokes and heart disease. Ephedra is currently under intense scrutiny by the FDA.

Take-Home Points

- Testosterone replacement therapy is indicated for men with low serum testosterone levels. Carefully consider which route of administration is preferable (transdermal or injection) and discuss this with your doctor.

- It is extremely important to have baseline liver function levels, prostate-specific antigen (PSA), and cholesterol measurements in conjunction with testosterone therapy.

- Many men who proceed with injection therapy can easily do this at home. It can dramatically save costs in the form of physician visits and injection costs as well.

- Herbs are powerful medications and should be taken in moderation.

- When you consult your physician, it is important to disclose the fact that you are taking herbs. Many patients usually don't mention it unless specifically asked.

Chapter 7
Medical Therapy

The most ideal situation for men with erectile dysfunction is to have a medication that can be taken by mouth just prior to sexual activities and would produce a great erection. This is every patient's and every physician's dream. Unfortunately, at the current time no such great therapy exists. There are, however, drugs and methods currently under study that will approach the ideal treatment. These will be discussed in chapter 10.

For thousands of years men have tried numerous compounds to stimulate erections. These range from rhinoceros horns, snake venom, and snake blood in the Orient. Such folk remedies have resulted in a tremendous decrease in the rhinoceros population but not a tremendous improvement in erections.

Currently, the most widely used oral therapy for erectile dysfunction is yohimbine. This drug is taken from the bark of a South American tree and acts as a weak blocker of the alpha receptor. It is widely available in health food stores and is advertised in the back pages of many men's magazines. Initial reports indicated some improvement in men, but it appeared that it was most effective in men who had psychological erectile dysfunction. Clinical studies show that yohimbine actually has minimal improvement in men with physiologic erectile dysfunction. It is generally administered orally in a dose of 5.4 mg three times a day and needs to be taken continuously. Additionally, it has side effects that include dizziness and headaches, and in my clinical experience, most men do not stay with this drug for long periods of time. It should not be used in men who have heart disease.

The only other drug currently available to treat erectile dysfunction is the antidepressant trazodone. It was originally found that men who took this drug for depression, had, as a side effect, priapism. This discovery led to its use by some as an oral drug for the treatment of erectile dysfunction because of trazodone's unique side effect. Various dosage regimens yield positive results. The general dosage is 50 mg three times a day. A major side effect is sedation. Again, this is not perfect therapy. Patients should be made aware that this is an antidepressant. I have had numerous calls from pharmacists and from angry patients, who have told me, "I didn't know that you thought I was depressed."

Topical Treatments

Another ideal treatment option is to have a compound that could be rubbed on the penis to produce an erection. This ideal compound would have no toxic side effects, would be safe for the partner, and would produce an erection that would last as long as desired. Unfortunately, this magical compound does not exist.

What is available is nitroglycerine ointment, an ointment used in the treatment of heart disease. It's primary use is for angina or chest pain, and it is the same drug that is placed under the tongue when patients have heart pain. Nitroglycerine is absorbed quickly, allows the coronary arteries to dilate or open, and allows oxygen to get to the heart muscle. It is quite effective for the treatment of angina. Studies regarding the use of nitroglycerine ointment on the penis have not been impressive. Some side effects include severe headaches, which are often seen in patients who use nitroglycerine for chest pain. Patients have also tried rubbing the drug minoxidil on the penis. This is the same medication used to produce hair growth. Studies on the use of minoxidil were not impressive; however, many patients have told me that this is a viable option.

Transurethral Therapy

Recently, the FDA approved alprostadil (MUSE), a small pellet that is administered in the urethra with good initial results (see Figure 7.1). The MUSE pellet has been found to be effective, and a large clinical study found that it did

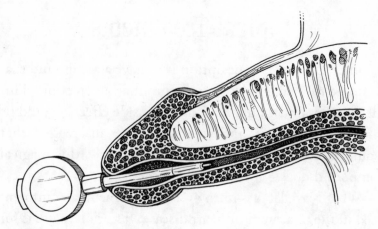

Figure 7.1. Insertion of the stem of the MUSE applicator into the urethra.
Vivus, Inc.

not have a great deal of side effects. The most common side effect was penile pain in roughly 36 percent of men who participated in the study. Urethral pain was reported in 13 percent of the men, and a small group of men had other side effects such as testicular discomfort, some urethral bleeding and spotting, and minor abrasions to the urethra. Also, low blood pressure occurred in about 3 percent of the patients. Overall, it was determined to be safe and effective and has a low incidence of priapism associated with it.

There are currently four dosage strengths available: 125, 250, 500, and 1,000 mcg; the urologist will determine the dose based on the patient's clinical history. I often prescribe the 500-mcg dose and will frequently go to 1,000. The onset of effect is roughly five to ten minutes and usually lasts from thirty minutes to an hour. It is not recommended for use more than once in a twenty-four-hour period. Patients also find that it works better with a ring-type device to prevent the drug from getting absorbed into the systemic circulation.

I also find that massaging the penis for several minutes increases the response.

Rare side effects do occur. One of the more unusual side effects involved a case where the MUSE pellet became caught in a female partner's mouth during oral sex and created an allergic reaction which necessitated a trip to the emergency room. For this reason, oral sex is not recommended when using the MUSE system. Aside from this, it is extremely easy to use and easy to learn as well.

Penile Injections

Prior to the advent of intracorporeal pharmacotherapy, or penile injections, penile prosthesis was the only thing other than drug therapy really available. The advent of penile injections began when a scientist working with dogs found that papaverine injected into the penis produced an erection.

The initial drug was papaverine, and this was then mixed with a drug called phentolamine. Papaverine was originally marketed for use in vascular surgery to dilate vessels and additionally was taken as an oral medication to act as a vaso dilator in people with lower extremity ischemia and people with vascular diseases of the legs. The off-label indication was used extensively throughout the 1980s. More papaverine was sold in the first year that this usage was discovered than had been sold in the prior thirty years.

Alprostadil, which was the manufactured version of prostaglandin E-1, proved to be effective as well. This drug caused relaxation of the corporal smooth muscle and produced an erection. It could be tolerated well and was sold for use in babies with heart abnormalities. The vials of alprostadil came in a highly concentrated form and were then diluted for use as penile injections. Prostaglandin by itself had a fairly high response rate, but when mixed with phentolamine and papaverine, its effectiveness was greatly increased.

In 1995, the Upjohn Company had alprostadil powder approved for use as a penile injection. The product, known as Caverject, comes as a dry powder and liquid is added to it at the time of use (see Figure 7.2). It originally came in 10- and 20-mcg vials. Recently, another unique formulation of alprostadil with an alpha-cyclo dextrin ring (called alprostadil alphadex) has been approved by the FDA for use. Manufactured by Schwarz Pharmaceuticals, this formulation tends to be more heat-stable and effective over a wide variety of doses, ranging up to 40 mcg. The vast majority of patients who use it achieve an excellent erection and high level of partner satisfaction.

Prior to the advent of these FDA-approved standardized dosage regimens, prostaglandin came in a diluted fashion, typically using up to 10 to 20 mcg per cc. Prostaglandin alone achieved a poor clinical response so Regitine was added (termed *bi-mix*). If this continued to fail, a third medication called phentolamine, termed *tri-mix*, was added. While each of these medications is FDA approved for different uses, their use either singly or in combination was not, so it was important to notify patients that these drugs were being used in an off-label manner.

I generally reserve the more exotic mixtures when the standard regimen fails. Some have advocated the use of an

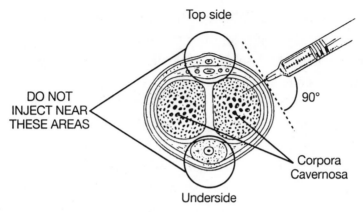

Figure 7.2. Penile injection therapy.
Pharmacia & Upjohn (Caverject® Sterile Solution)

additional drug atropine, which can speed up the heart rate and also improve erections as well. Because it has more potential for side effects it is generally not recommended. Finally, a plant compound called Forskolin (discussed in chapter 8), a derivative of an herb found in the Indian subcontinent, can also help to improve erections and is especially useful in men who do not respond to the standard tri-mix regimen.

The actual technique of penile injections involves the use of a fine 29 or 30 gauge needle and 1-cc syringe, which is the same type of syringe that diabetics use for insulin, to inject as small a volume of fluid as possible. I generally like the patients to inject the 10:00 and the 2:00 position in the sides of the penis.

The needle is placed in a perpendicular fashion to inject the entire contents of the syringe. It is not necessary to get a return of blood in the needle. Direct pressure should be applied over the injection site for several minutes. If the patient is on blood thinners such as Coumadin or aspirin, pressure is applied to the injection site for an additional

B.F. was a sixty-five-year-old with erectile dysfunction. He had long-standing diabetes and had been
recommended to use penile injections. He came to the
emergency room with priapism because he had an
erection for more than twelve hours. He had given
himself six injections in the preceding twelve hours.
These injections were all unrelated to each other, and
they were with six different partners. We were able to
reduce the erection with irrigation of the penis with
drugs to reduce the priapism.

period. Consent should always be obtained prior to an injection program to clearly document that this procedure is not
without risks.

I always start penile injection therapy in the office with
careful instructions and closely follow the patient. This technique appears deceptively simple, but it is not without
numerous complications and side effects. Patients are at risk
for scarring if the procedure is not performed correctly, and
as a consequence of scarring, patients can also develop angulation and a variant of Peyronie's disease.

There are minimal contraindications to treatment with
pharmacological intercavernosal injections. The major
contraindication would be an allergy to prostaglandin,
papaverine, or regitine. Patients who are at risk for
priapism should be carefully counseled as well. Additionally,
patients on anticoagulants for conditions that require thinning of the blood are advised to put extra pressure on the
penis after an injection.

I usually recommend using the injections no more than

three times per week. Although patients have used them two or three times per day, I do not recommend this. I also do not recommend an additional injection if the first response is not complete. It is extremely important not to share this medication with your friends as this has happened on occasion.

Complications

Pain is not an infrequent complication of intercavernosal injection therapy, particularly with prostaglandin. The pain tends to be an aching sensation, but most patients are able to tolerate it. Very few patients drop out of a pharmocologic erection program because of pain. A few men feel that the pain is disabling to their erections, so I recommend taking two extra-strength Tylenol tablets one hour before anticipated injection and relations. This generally works well. We are not sure why men develop pain, although it tends to be more common with prostaglandin than with the other agents.

The most dreaded complication of intracorporal penile injections is a prolonged erection and priapism. Prolonged erections and priapism can result from any single drug or any combination of drugs. Any erection greater than two hours duration is defined as prolonged, and priapism is when an erection lasts longer than four hours. There is no absolute definition of a prolonged erection or priapism, but any man who has used a penile injection and has an erection that lasts for more than two hours should consider immediate medical attention. After a period of two hours, the penis begins to develop a low oxygen state and can begin to develop scarring and ultimately the loss of corporal smooth muscle.

B.C. was a fifty-one-year-old man who was on a stable course of prostaglandin injections for his erectile dysfunction. It worked quite well for him, but another man, his friend, came to the emergency room with priapism. On careful questioning, it turned out that B.C. had given him the injections as well as instruction. Although this man had no erectile dysfunction, he thought it would augment his functioning and used the injection. This resulted in priapism for more than six hours.

I instruct all my patients to have pseudoephedrine on hand and to take a single tablet if their erection isn't gone within an hour. If this is unsuccessful, terbutaline, a drug used for the treatment of asthma has been successful in abating most prolonged erections. However, if a man truly begins to develop priapism, it is important to get treatment within three to four hours. The first treatment option is to irrigate the penis and aspirate the old blood out. (This is discussed in chapter 5 on priapism.) Simply removing the blood and oxygenating the tissues with fresh blood is sometimes all that is necessary. If, however, it is a fairly resistant erection and returns, I then use a mixture of phenylephrine. Blood pressure and heart rate must be carefully monitored as cases of cardiac problems have been related to these medications as well.

Another worrisome complication is scarring. All drugs have different cases of scarring. Prostaglandin tends to have the lowest instance of scarring, and some studies indicate that prostaglandin may actually protect the corporal smooth muscle from the development of scarring related to age. Papaverine has been associated with the most degree of scarring. This was initially thought to be related to the pH of the solution, and the occurrecne is nearly 100 percent in some cases. Rare long-term side effects of scarring include curvature, similar to Peyronie's disease. Severe scarring may require a straightening procedure, much like the treatment for Peyronie's disease.

One of the benefits of intracavernosal injections is an overall improvement in erections. Many men report that their erections are actually better for several episodes of intercourse after a single penile injection and, therefore, will tend to use it infrequently.

There is also a fairly high dropout rate from penile injections. Reasons include fear of the needle and medication costs. Although the treatment produces an excellent erection, it is not the ideal panacea and has drawbacks: the needle, the need for partner preparation, and frankly, the loss of spontaneity. This is probably the number one complaint from patients and their partners.

Insurance and Erectile Dysfunction

This is one of the more important aspects of the book. In this section I will discuss the correct coding of the diagnosis and any treatments. If these are not coded correctly, they will not be reimbursed. Although it is difficult to keep up with the many coding changes that occur, unfortunately, coding is how we live and die in medicine in the nineties. Each diagnosis is given a specific code, and each treatment option is given a specific code. These codes are used to support each other to be sure of what is termed a "medical necessity." The Health Care Financing Administration has developed a national policy that specifically addresses the diagnosis and treatment of erectile dysfunction.

> Program payment may be made for diagnosis and treatment of sexual impotence. Impotence is the failure of a body part for which the diagnosis, and frequently the treatment, require medical expertise. Depending on the cause of the condition, treatment may be surgical, e.g. implantation of a penile pros-thesis, or nonsurgical, e.g. medical or psychotherapeutic treatment. Since causes and therefore appropriate treatments vary, if abuse is suspected it may be necessary to request documentation of appropriateness in individual cases. If treatment is furnished to patients (other than hospital patients) in connection with a mental condition, apply the psychiatric service limitation described in Medicare Carriers Manual #2470.

It's unfortunate that this is a fairly vague national policy, and as the Health Care Financing Administration increases its fraud division, we will expect to see more investigation into questionable practices. It is important for patients to know that their treatment is appropriate so that they are not left with a treatment option that is not reimbursed or one that results in insurance problems.

Most insurance carriers have or will soon adopt Medicare policies. An additional caveat is that erectile dysfunction must have existed continuously for at least six months to qualify for assessment or treatment. With the advent and FDA approval of the self-administered urethral suppository

(MUSE), this is added to previously available regimens of penile injections, vacuum erection devices, and penile prostheses. Medicare feels that these treatments are effective, and the treatment option is determined both by the patient's physician and the patient themselves. They further state that duplex ultrasound is an indicated procedure if used in consideration of vascular surgery in men younger than thirty who have had a fractured penis or trauma.

Medicare states that if psychiatric elements predominate in the diagnosis, then psychotherapy may be necessary. A nocturnal penile tumescence study would confirm this. They also note that if Peyronie's disease causes painful erections, surgical correction may be indicated. Interestingly, in men over fifty years of age, Medicare feels that the current treatments are beneficial for all types of erectile dysfunction and that the need for extensive laboratory testing, X ray, or ultrasound studies beyond the basic history and physical examination is lacking. Therefore, elaborate radiographic or physiologic or neurologic testing is not covered because Medicare does not feel it has a role in determining the type of therapy.

The Health Care Financing Administration guidelines also state that medications are not Medicare covered, including the MUSE, Caverject, and Edex because they are self-administered drugs given in the office for instruction, demonstration, or titration purposes. The only thing that is truly covered is the careful history and physical examination and appropriate radiographic and laboratory testing. To perform this testing, the history and physical must support the need for appropriate laboratory or radiographic testing. Drugs are not covered, although a few private insurance plans do cover drugs. Testosterone replacement is also a currently non-covered service.

If there are any questions with regards to what is reimbursed, consult your physician prior to undergoing the test, as this will help avoid any subsequent problems.

Take-Home Points

- Before having an invasive procedure be sure it is covered. Precertification does not guarantee payment.
- Avoid "erection shops" where every patient is given every test.
- Always question any billing discrepancies.

Chapter 8

Nonsurgical Treatments

Vacuum Erection Devices

Vacuum erection devices (VEDs) are not a new treatment for erectile dysfunction; this treatment dates back to the last century. Before the advent of modern VEDs, the majority of these devices were found in the back of men's magazines and were sold as penis enlargers. Parts associated with these devices were not standardized, and they were certainly not part of the mainstream treatment of erectile dysfunction. Most clinicians tended to avoid them because of their lack of familiarity with the devices and the shortage of peer-reviewed medical literature about them. Only until the National Institutes of Health Consensus Conference on Erectile Dysfunction took place did VEDs become a reasonable option for the treatment of erectile dysfunction. Vacuum devices are currently one of the most popular treatments utilized in my practice. This device is useful for all patients suffering from erectile dysfunction, and when the patient wants to participate in goal-directed therapy, it's a reasonable alternative to surgery.

In goal-directed therapy, we know that despite the workup for erectile dysfunction, treatment options will always be the same, and many people would rather proceed with the treatment than a costly workup that won't really change the treatment option.

The Device

Vacuum erection devices (VEDs) and their component parts are all of different quality (see Figure 8.1). The basic unit of vacuum erection devices is the cylinder, which is a clear plastic sleeve that fits over the penis. The person fitting the cylinder should be able to actually visualize the penis. This is to avoid the complications of bleeding, hematomas, or bruises on the shaft of the penis. The cylinder must be sized correctly, especially for men who have too short or too long a penis. If the cylinder does not fit properly, the vacuum erection device is ineffective. So, many manufacturers have gotten around this by providing a plastic insert to narrow the opening that the penis sits in, allowing the patient to achieve a tighter seal. The tighter seal provides more suction and prevents the scrotum from getting sucked into the tube and making it uncomfortable.

The cylinder is then connected to a pump that has a quick-release valve. The pump can be one of two types; it can be either one-handed or two-handed. There is really no advantage or disadvantage to either one; it is simply a matter of patient preference. Battery-operated pumps are also available. I find that these are more useful in patients with arthritis or hand problems who may have difficulty pumping and manipulating the ring at the same time. In any event, it is important to limit the negative pressure to less than 350 mm of mercury. If this is not the case, many patients will complain of pain.

The third component of the VED is the tension ring. After the erection is achieved with the vacuum device, the tension ring constricts the venous return of the penis and allows the erection to be maintained. A whole host of different rings are available. I have had patients tell me they use the rubber band off the newspaper with strings tied to it as a tension ring. Rings come in several sizes and should be made of material that cannot be broken down by silicone-based lubricating jelly. Some of the better rings have a notch to allow the ejaculate to spurt forward. The major problem with rings is that they can sometimes break, and this necessitates replacing the rings. Rings can also wear out with repeated usage.

The most important part of the VED is the instruction and training that goes with the device itself. Many physicians will often hand the patient a vacuum erection device with a video without demonstrating the device. I strongly feel it is important to demonstrate the VED to the patient and help troubleshoot some of its problems. It is also important to discuss the risk factors with the patient and review who will not be a good candidate for a VED. Frequently, people prefer to move right to the treatment option and avoid the diagnostic phase, although for these people, the VED is still a reasonable option.

After the patient has assembled the device, a lubricant is used to obtain a better seal to the skin at the base of the penis. Some of the problems patients have had include difficulty obtaining a tight seal due to excessive pubic hair. In these situations, patients shave the hair at the base of the penis and along the area where the scrotum comes in contact with the penis. It is also important to keep the scrotum out of the way to prevent it from being sucked up when the negative pressure is being applied to the penis.

Once the patient has achieved a rigid erection, the tension ring, which has been preloaded against the cylinder, is released and pushed on the penis. Lubrication facilitates this. The vacuum is then released by the quick-release valve. When training the patient to use the VED it is important to explain that it will not result in the normal feel of a rock-hard erection. The penis tends to be more purplish in color and can actually be cold as well. Patients' sexual partners sometimes complain about the cold feeling, and in some instances, patients discontinue use of the VED because of the cold sensation. I recommend wrapping a warm, moist towel around the penis prior to penetration or using a warming lubrication jelly to avoid this problem. Some patients complain of pain with maximum inflation of the penis. In this case, I have them train themselves with the device to become comfortable with the different levels of engorgement.

Side effects that have been reported include numbness, difficulty with orgasm, and decrease in the force of the ejaculate, as well as bruising and swelling of the penis. VEDs have worked in patients who have had prostheses removed

J.F. was a sixty-five-year-old man who had a placement of a penile prosthesis. The device was removed
following operative complications. Because of
substantial scarring, he was not a candidate for an
additional device. He was trained in the technique of
a vacuum erection device, and by using two tension
bands, he was able to maintain enough erection for
vaginal penetration. While it was not an excellent
erection, it was certainly adequate for intercourse, and
he was pleased.

and who use these devices in addition to having a penile
prosthesis. These men usually want additional glans
tumescence, and this is the reason they use it. Patients also
choose vacuum devices in conjunction with penile injections. Patients even use a VED to help stimulate erections
without needing the ring for intercourse. Men with a venous
leak have used the tension ring to help maintain the erection. They have no trouble achieving erection, but the ring
helps trap the blood in the penis and prevent the leakage
that causes the sudden loss of erection.

A vacuum erection device does not produce an erection
as solid as when you were eighteen years old. Most patients
who use a VED achieve tumescence but really don't have the
rigidity that they were used to. On a 10 point scale, most
patients report an erection between 7 and 9 with a VED.
This means that some buckling occurs with penetration, but
the satisfaction rate with VEDs is high. The vast majority
of patients are pleased with the device, and they are pleased
that they are now able to have intercourse.

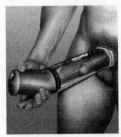

1. Place flaccid penis in cylinder.

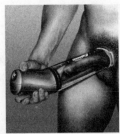

2. Create negative pressure to achieve vascular engorgement

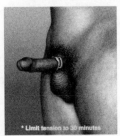

3. Apply tension to maintain rigidity and engorgement. (limit tension to 30 minutes.)

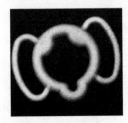

4. Pressure Point™ tension ring.

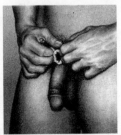

5. Remove tension ring. Penis returns to flaccid state.

Figure 8.1. Vacuum erection device.
Osbon Medical Systems

In my experience, the VEDs tend to be more useful for the older patient. Many of the worries that men have had before they became comfortable with the device quickly become less of a problem. Some initial worries include the length of time it takes to set up the device. Reports in the literature say that the average patient, once comfortable with the device, can achieve an erection reasonable for intercourse within two minutes. Many men use the device and the inflation of their penis as part of foreplay. Men who choose VEDs

Y.M. was a forty-five-year-old man who was involved in a severe accident at work resulting in loss of sensation and blood flow to his penis. He tried numerous options, but eventually settled on a penile prosthesis. He found out, however, that his glans did not become engorged, and this made intercourse unsatisfactory. By the use of the penile implant plus the vacuum erection device, he was able to restore the length of his penis that was present before the injury and allow the glans to become much larger and increase friction, thereby making intercourse more satisfactory.

in my experience tend to have long-term, stable relationships and are generally older.

Reimbursement Issues

Medicare usually covers vacuum erection devices with the use of the appropriate code for erectile dysfunction and an additional code that indicates the reason for the erectile dysfunction. Many private insurance companies require pre-certification prior to approval. Again, as with penile implants, I recommend that this process be done prior to receiving the implant to be sure that the full benefits are realized. Most manufacturers of VEDs have toll-free numbers for twenty-four-hour consultation by trained professional staff, and provide in-office training demonstrations for individual patients.

The cost of VEDs is extremely variable. They range from less than $100 to $500 for the premium devices. The old adage, "You get what you pay for" is true. The more premium devices tend to give better service and a better product. Since third-party pairs routinely reimburse the cost of the least expensive device, it is up to the patient to provide the cost difference. Patients will generally choose the more expensive device because of reliability and because of the company's policies.

Weights

Penile weights are not a new concept. Penile weights date back many thousands of years when they had been utilized by both African and Indian tribes from puberty onward to lengthen the penis. These are generally a system of increasingly heavier weights that are placed on the penis and left on for fairly long periods of time. They can result in an elongated penis.

There are no prescriptive penile weights. The actual medical use of these is after a suspensory ligament is cut or after a penile lengthening procedure. These weights are then recommended to prevent scarring. There are numerous novelty devices on the market. These weight-training systems are available from 2- to 3-pound weights that are hung via a small snare on the head of the penis. A more inexpensive device can be used that hooks over the head of the penis and uses elastic bands to strap to the ankle. Again these are not really recommended in a conventional setting, but only for men who have had prior surgery and wish to prevent scarring after a penile lengthening procedure.

Rings

Penile rings are also known as "cock rings." These are an ancient method to produce constriction of the penis causing the penis to enlarge somewhat. These rings have been made of numerous materials, including rubber, leather, Velcro, and vinyl. Metal rings are also used, but are exceedingly difficult to move and can cause massive swelling of the penis. Again, these are sold as novelty items and are not medically recommended except as part of a vacuum erection device. These rings are made of surgical-grade latex that have bands on both sides to allow easy removal. They are also not tight enough to cause damage to the penis.

Penile rings are one of the best first-line techniques for men with venous leak problems. The newest device available is the Actis Venous Flow Controller, which is specifically designed to enhance erections by decreasing the blood return from the penis. It has an adjustable loop placed around the base of the penis with a slide to easily increase or decrease tension. It allows blood to continue to flow in the penis via the cavernosal artery but impedes the blood to the surface of the penis and produces quite a bit of increased engorgement of the glans penis (see Figure 8.2). I only recommend it to patients who have difficulty maintaining erections because of a venous leak.

The device is simple to use. It is stretched over the head

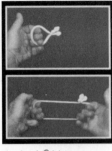

1. Actis® Venous Flow Controller.

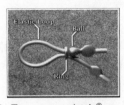

2. To prepare Actis®, grasp loop of Actis® device. (Note: The end of the tubing with the belt is on top.) With the other hand, grasp loop next to the O-ring and stretch.

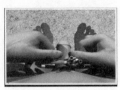

3. Place end of the penis through the stretched loop and slide Actis® device over shaft of the penis until it is positioned around the base.

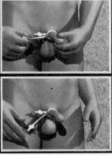

4. Grasp finger grip (lower end) of tubing without the ball. Pull horizontally away from the penis until snug. Ends of the tubing should be located on the side of the shaft of the penis with ball on top.

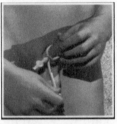

5. Grasp fingergrip on the end of tubing without the ball and pull down. The Actis® device should be tight enough to keep blood from leaving the penis.

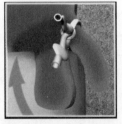

6. If erection is not rigid enough, masage the perineum to push more blood into the penis.

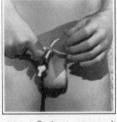

7. The Actis® device may be loosened by pulling up on the end of the tubing with the ball.

Figure 8.2. Actis® Venous Flow Controller
Vivus, Inc.

of the penis and placed at the base of the shaft, so that the loop encircles the base of the penis. The portion of the tubing with the ball end is placed toward the topside of the penis, and then the device is snugged down. It is tight enough to keep the blood from leaving the penis, but it does not and should not cause pain. After intercourse the device may be loosened or removed. This device is widely available in physicians' offices, but it is not for patients who have a latex allergy or any penile abnormalities in regards to shape. I also recommend using it for less than thirty minutes only. If the tension is enough to cause pain, it is too much. The only side effects are some redness at the site of the ring and a prolonged erection. This is the only medical-grade ring device that is available, and it is recommended on a fairly regular basis.

Take-Home Points

- Vacuum erection devices (VEDs) are a reasonable choice for the management of erectile dysfunction.

- It is important to have the device pre-certified by your insurance company to be sure that they will reimburse for the cost of the device.

- Be sure to choose a device that has a generous return policy, so if mechanical malfunction were to take place, it can be returned for replacement or a refund.

- The Actis device is useful in men with venous leakage.

- Penile weights are novelty items at best and dangerous unless used in a monitored postoperative setting.

Chapter 9

Surgery: Penile Prosthesis and Enlargement

Penile Prosthesis

Penile prosthesis in the right patient is a blessing, but in a poorly selected patient it is a nightmare. Prosthetic implants have been available since the seventies. Unfortunately, the early devices were plagued with problems such as malfunction, infection, and erosion. For these reasons they received a bad reputation.

Deciding to have a penile prosthesis is probably one of the most difficult for a man. There are many factors that need to be taken into account by both the patient and the implanting surgeon. My personal feeling regarding penile implants is that it is truly the last resort. The candidate for a penile implant typically has had the full diagnostic workup indicating no other options and a full therapeutic attempt has been made, including vacuum erection devices and penile injections.

Indications

The indications for a penile implant are men with severe organic erectile dysfunction who have no other treatment options. These are typically men with diabetes in whom the vacuum erection device fails to provide satisfactory erection or maintain the rigidity required for penetration. The physician must carefully discuss the prosthesis device with both the patient and the patient's sexual partner as it is imperative that the sexual partner be in full agreement with the need and desire for a penile implant.

Relatively less stringent indications include men who, for a variety of reasons, don't want to give themselves penile injections or for whom injections do not work. After the decision has been made to proceed with the penile implant, it is important to find an experienced implanting surgeon.

Although many urologists in training have some working knowledge of penile implants, only a surgeon who regularly performs this procedure or who has the most experience confronting difficult situations when complications arise should do the implant. It is also important to ascertain how many of the devices the surgeon has done. At least six to twelve procedures per year maintains clinical competence in this arena. If a surgeon does this procedure infrequently, the patient should ask for names of other surgeons at a referral center. Many of these names are well known to the urologic community and can even be obtained by consulting the Internet.

The next step is to decide on the type of device to choose. A vast array of these devices exist, so a good framework to begin with is to ask whether you want a semi-rigid or malleable prosthesis or an inflatable device (see Figures 9.1 to 9.7).

Semi-Rigid and Malleable Prostheses

Semi-rigid prostheses are usually a variation of the original Small-Carrion model, which was one of the original semi-rigid prostheses. The implanting procedure consists of a series of incisions made in the corporal body, and the corporal body is then gently dilated with a series of graded dilators to enlarge the cavity, which is carefully measured. The original Small-Carrion device was available in numerous sizes and was tapered to fit into the corporal body. These paired rods allowed moderate rigidity and, in certain situations, the glans retained the ability to become tumescent, allowing satisfactory intercourse. Certainly it didn't produce as rigid an erection as a normal erection, but it was suitable and patient satisfaction rate was reasonable.

Diameter was a problem with the original devices. In a person with an unusually large or small penis, these devices were poor options. The mechanical reliability of these devices has been excellent. The major drawbacks are the degree of rigidity and some more unusual complications, such as erosion of the device into the urethra. This is not typical, but it has occurred in people with spinal cord injuries who have decreased sensation.

In preparation for the device, the candidate should have no preexisting difficulties that will cause complications. If you have difficulty urinating initially, for instance, having a constantly-erect penis will not aid it. Unfortunately, when the prosthesis is in place, it makes access to the prostate from a transurethral approach difficult and sometimes impossible. This necessitates cutting a hole in the urethra at the base of the penis to allow access to the prostate. This is certainly not an ideal situation.

One of the newer malleable devices is the Duraphase penile prosthesis, a malleable device that has one distinct advantage over the semi-rigid devices: it can be bended, allowing it to be concealed. This device is a series of segments, much like a centipede, strung on a tough, thickened cable that sit upon each other. You can bend it down, but when you straighten the segments, they tend to sit upon each other and allow axial rigidity. The satisfaction rate with this device has been excellent. It is an especially good device in men with Peyronie's disease, as it allows not only the ability to straighten the penis, but to provide a satisfactory erection for penetration. One keynote with regard to the semi-rigid and malleable devices is penile length. Men with greater-than-average size penises do not consistently have good results, nor do men with smaller-than-average penises. Extremes on both ends of the spectrum do not constitute a great number of men, but size is something that should be considered between the patient and the implanting surgeon.

Inflatable Devices

The next series of devices are self-contained inflatable penile prostheses. These prostheses consist of a pair of cylinders much like the malleable devices, but they have an internal balloon that, by pumping the head, allows fluid to transfer to an outer shape and create rigidity. These devices are not as popular as the true three-piece inflatable devices, and the initial success is excellent, but many of the patients are dissatisfied because it is somewhat difficult to manipulate and because of problems with the device itself. They are relatively simple to put in, but again, these are not really meant for patients with large or small penises. One important point is that over the years, repeated inflation and deflation can cause a weakening of the flexion points of the penis-scrotal junction and can actually cause erosion.

There are a number of two-piece inflatable penile prostheses that consist of two cylinders and one pump. These are made by two U.S. manufacturers: American Medical Systems and Mentor. One fault of these devices is the fairly large sized reservoir that is placed in the scrotum. This can be somewhat uncomfortable for men with small scrotums and can be quite noticeable in some situations, especially in men who are thin or who have relatively small penises and scrotums.

Finally, the multiple-component inflatables, or the three-piece prostheses, are probably the most popular inflatable devices. These consist of the paired cylinders, a pump, and a reservoir in a separate location. They are also the most expensive of all the prostheses and the most difficult to implant so they are not for the occasional implant surgeon.

American Medical Systems makes the widest variety and produces a number of different cylinders that may be used. Many of the cylinders are developed for very different situations, including a scarred corporal body in patients who have had infections or who have had prior penile implants. One very important rule in patients who have had multiple-

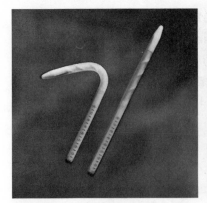

Figure 9.1. Acu-Form penile implant.
Mentor

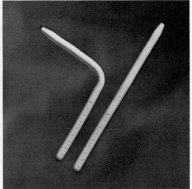

Figure 9.2. Malleable penile implant.
Mentor

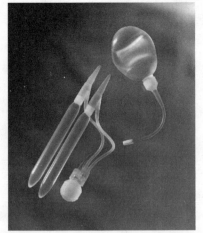

Figure 9.3. Alpha 1 Narrow Base implant.
Mentor

component penile prostheses: Never switch these patients to a malleable rod. They invariably will be unhappy, because these rods do not come close to being as lifelike an erection as can be obtained with a multipiece inflatable device.

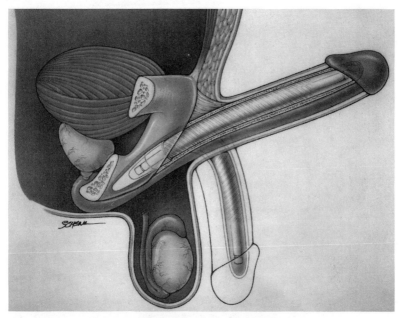

Figure 9.4. Malleable 650™ penile prosthesis.
Courtesy of American Medical Systems, Inc., Minnetonka, Minnesota. Illustration by Michael Schenk.

After one chooses the type of device, the next major decision is the type of incision used to implant the device. A semi-rigid or malleable prostheses can be implanted through numerous incisions, including the peno-scrotal incision, sub-cronal incision, and the perineal incision. The two-piece prostheses can be implanted in the peno-scrotal operation. The three-piece prostheses is implanted in two fashions: One is the infra-pubic incision, which is made above the penis. This seems to be what most surgeons in the United States tend to use because of the relative ease of placing the reservoir. The other is the peno-scrotal incision.

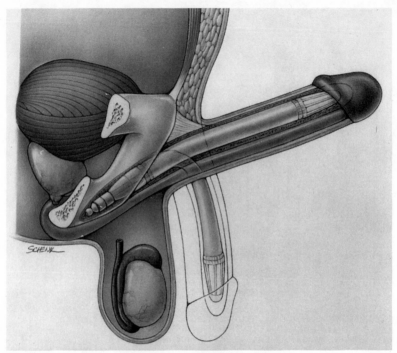

Figure 9.5. Dynaflex™ penile prosthesis.
Courtesy of American Medical Systems, Inc., Minnetonka, Minnesota. Illustration by Michael Schenk.

Complications

Perhaps the most difficult part of penile prostheses is complications. Complications can occur at any phase of the procedure. Even the most experienced implant surgeons encounter complications. The difference in the experience is how these complications are managed. This is the reason you should choose an experienced implant surgeon.

The most dreaded complication of implant surgery is infection. The most common infecting organism is *Staphylococcus epidermis*, an organism that typically colonizes the skin and when it infects the prosthesis, the results can be disastrous. Meticulous scrubbing of the genitalia for

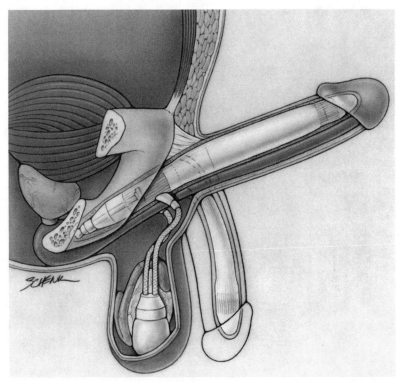

Figure 9.6. Ambicor® penile prosthesis.
Courtesy of American Medical Systems, Inc., Minnetonka, Minnesota. Illustration by Michael Schenk.

several weeks before the operation with antibacterial scrub is necessary. Broad-spectrum antibiotics are given before the surgery and continue after the surgery. Everything possible is done to prevent infections. Unfortunately, infections still can and do occur. Typically, patients with diabetes are at a greater risk for infections. It was erroneously thought that diabetes and poor control predisposed patients to recurrent infections, however, this was never definitively proven.

Another postsurgical complication is uncontrolled bleeding that results in hematoma, or a collection of blood beneath the tissue. This is typically self-limiting, but

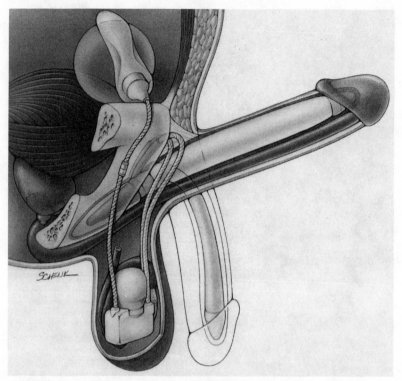

Figure 9.7. 700 Ultrex™ Plus penile prosthesis.
Courtesy of American Medical Systems, Inc., Minnetonka, Minnesota. Illustration by Michael Schenk.

sometimes it means a reoperation, which exposes the prosthesis to more risk of infection. Other acute postoperative
problems are related to the surgical procedure or the anesthetic, such as breathing problems and heart attacks. For this
reason, it is important to do a thorough preoperative evaluation and address these problems in a prospective manner.

Scar tissue is a common complication of the operation.
When scar tissue occurs, it can create a capsule and prevent
the cylinders from totally expanding. Also, pain is expected
after a surgical procedure, but pain after a certain period of
time may be the earliest sign of an infection. Some diabetic

patients may develop pain that is difficult to control and may last for several months. Some patients will even notice a decreased sensitivity in the penis. This typically improves because the nerves that are involved with sensation at the head of the penis are far enough away from the operative incisions used to implant the device.

One good way to avoid complications is to do a careful evaluation of the patient's manual dexterity. A patient who has limited function of the hands should not be recommended for a three-piece device that is difficult to inflate and deflate. Also, the patient with an extremely large penis would be a poor candidate for the semi-rigid type of device, as would a patient with a small penis. The best device for men with either very large or small penises is the three-piece inflatable device.

Scarring in the corporal bodies may also be found at the time of the implant. Scar tissue can make it difficult to dilate the corporal body and can make placement of a prosthetic cylinder extremely difficult. Patients who are at risk for this include those who have had a previous penile implant, infection, or trauma to the penis. Patients who have priapism can be the most difficult on which to perform implant procedures. Patients with Peyronie's disease can also be difficult to work on. The important key is to select an area that has never had either infection or scarring. Inside the penis the corporal bodies are paired cylinders that split as the penis comes closer to the body. Sometimes during the implantation, it is possible to perforate one of the corporal bodies and place the dilator on the other side. This phenomenon is known as a *crural crossover*, which occurs when both the proximal, or the parts that are close to the body, are present in the same corporal body. This can happen despite careful surgical practice. When the prosthesis is placed, the dilator is left in to allow the surgeon to develop a plane in the other body, avoiding this complication.

Other problems include perforation of the corporal body. Typically, the corporal body is a thickened, tough membrane and is resistant to the passage of the metal dilators, or saunds. However, patients who have had radiation therapy are predisposed to perforation since radiation results in thinning of the tissues. This can occur at either end of the corporal body. When it happens close to the body it can be fixed by sewing a thickened, tough material to the end of the prosthesis to fix it. When it happens toward the end of the penis and the metal dilator perforates into the urethra, this can be a potentially disastrous situation as it exposes the prosthesis to contamination by bacteria found in the urethra. In this situation, it is usually appropriate not to place the cylinder but to wait two months for the penis and the urethra to heal before a repeat attempt at insertion is made. If the cylinder has been placed on one side, it is appropriate to leave it in order to allow the penis to maintain its length. However, a patient will rarely be happy with the single cylinder.

Incorrect sizing of the implant can produce further problems. It is important to choose the right size cylinder, especially in patients with a malleable device. Too long of a cylinder can cause pain and deformity; too short of a cylinder can cause a deformity in which the tip of the penis is floppy. When using a three-piece multi-component device, such as the AMS 700 with ultrex-type cylinders (see Figure 9.7), these cylinders are downsized because the ultrex can expand longer than the corporal body and thus create a so-called S-shaped deformity. For patients who have smaller penises or severely scarred penises, a non-expanding cylinder called the CX cylinder helps take care of this problem. The downside of this is that it tends not to produce the girth that some patients prefer.

One of the more unusual problems we see with three-piece devices is auto-inflation. Auto-inflation is a spontaneous inflation of the device that occurs with heavy activity like lifting or bending. This is because increased pressure from such activities causes the fluid to be pushed from the reservoir through the pump into the cylinders. To avoid this, it's important to be sure that the cavity in which the reservoir sits is adequate enough to hold the volume and is not scarred. The best way to minimize auto-inflation is to make an adequate pocket for the reservoir. I tell patients to keep the penile implant completely deflated so that the reservoir heals in its fully expanded capacity. If a lot of fluid is transferred into the penis, a scar will develop around it, and this will prevent maximum inflation and can predispose one to auto-inflation. It is also important to do a back pressure test to make sure the prosthesis is not receiving too much pressure from the over-full reservoir. Despite all these attempts, auto-inflation can and does occur, so patients should be informed of this possibility.

Other problems with three-piece devices include aneurysms or a bulging of the cylinder. Prostheses manufacturers have made numerous attempts to avoid this, using both Gore-Tex and Dacron. I have actually seen a case where vigorous sexual intercourse resulted in a sudden aneurysm formation.

Erosion may also happen both to the corporal body into

the subcutaneous tissue and into the urethra. When this happens, it is usually a simple matter to expose the area that is eroded and to oversew this area with a suture. This procedure is called a *disto corporoplasty*. One of the more difficult problems is erosion of the penile implant into the urethra. This is typically a disastrous situation and needs immediate attention. Although erosion is unusual in patients who are neurologically intact, it is more common in patients who have spinal cord injuries or severe diabetes. As the penile prosthesis approaches the head of the penis there is a relatively narrow space in the urethra. A urethral catheter in diabetics or spinal cord injury patients can predispose them to erosion, resulting in a decrease in blood flow and bacterial colonization. The diagnosis is fairly simple: One needs merely to examine the penis to make the diagnosis. It is usually quite obvious. The treatment is to remove the prosthesis. Other rare complications are erosion of the reservoir into the bowel contents, but again, this is more common in patients who have had prior radiotherapy, which predisposes the tissues to being thinner and more susceptible to problems.

Other extremely rare occurrences include erosion of the penile prosthesis into a bedsore. Patients who have neurologic abnormalities tend to develop bedsores from sitting in one position for a long time. The penile prosthesis can erode into this massive infection. Again, the treatment is removal. Unfortunately, penile prostheses are also associated with a significant amount of malpractice.

Part of the controversy about penile implants includes silicone. Tremendous controversy surrounds the use of silicone, and it is important to realize that silicone coats the prosthesis. The use of silicone in the genitourinary system has had widespread popularity for many years, and numerous articles support the safety of these devices. However, the general public is often unaware that the use of silicone expands widely beyond the use in surgically implanted devices and includes coating of needles, nipples, and other everyday products.

Again the most important part of penile implants is to be sure that you have had a proper workup and full consent with regard to the penile implant including an extensive review of the risks and benefits discussed above. Most people who have penile implants are satisfied with them and would absolutely choose to do it again.

Penis Enlargement

I am asked on an almost daily basis if it is possible to enlarge the penis. My answer is always the same: If I could enlarge the penis, *I* would have a large penis. Before discussing penile enlargements, it is important to have an understanding of a normal-size penis. Unfortunately, there is no consensus on what constitutes a normal-sized penis.

Generally speaking, an adequate penis size is one that allows penetration of the vagina sufficient enough to permit fertilization and the ability to stand upright to urinate. When these two criteria are met, the penis is a normal length. The controversy that surrounds penile lengthening is tremendous. There are men who focus their entire lives on worrying about the length of their penis. Men have come to my office so upset that they are unable to function because of worries about penile size.

Much of the myth that surrounds penile length is exactly that, *myth*. There are tremendous differences in the measurement between the flaccid and the erect length. One common fallacy is that flaccid length can be a predictor of the erect length, and vice versa. This is not true. It is important to measure the penis with a full erection in a standardized fashion. The method we utilize is to place a rigid ruler on the dorsum (top) of the penis between the body and the tip of the glans. It is very important not to include the foreskin, especially in men who have a droopy, elongated foreskin. One should also avoid including as much of the superficial fat as possible.

In a busy urologic practice, I would say that the average penis is somewhere between 5 and 6 inches long. The only real indication for surgery to correct penile size is for people who have a true micropenis. These are typically children, and the medical definition for this patient is that when the penis is stretched, it measures more than 2.5 standard deviations below the mean for the given age. This is a very rare problem and usually has a hormonal cause.

This controversy surrounding the procedure arose because a very small group of urologists opened penile-lengthening clinics in certain states. The parent organization of most urologists, the American Urologic Association (AUA) discussed this issue in their 1994 national meeting. They found no justification for trying to augment either the girth or length of the penis.

Remember that the amount of body fat dictates the length of the penis. The general rule of thumb is that for every 30 pounds over ideal body weight, one can expect to lose roughly an inch of penile length. While this can be variable, it is extremely rare to see a large penis in a morbidly obese man, and the converse is usually true as well.

Men seeking penile enlargement must be aware of several facts. There is no standardized treatment, and there are no standardized results. The complication rate for this particular type of operation is tremendous if it is not done by highly experienced hands. Physicians who do this type of operation claim they can actually increase the penis from one to three inches in length. They also claim the average gain is two inches. This unfortunately has not been proven yet. Several procedures are currently available, and these are based on the patient's individual anatomy.

Surgical Procedures for Length

One procedure involves the release of the suspensory ligament. The suspensory ligament of the penis is a thick ligament that extends from the base of the abdominal muscles along the bone called the *symphysis*. It is the structure that anchors the penis to the body. Dividing this suspensory ligament can give the appearance of an increase in penile length. What it actually does is to destabilize it during penetration. Suspensory ligament cuts can cause the penis to retract and become shortened postoperatively. To prevent this, penile weights are utilized to allow the penis to heal in the new position without the suspensory ligament. Penile weights are not medical devices, but there are numerous types available.

Another procedure to give the appearance of penile lengthening is to move the web of tissue that extends from the scrotum to the shaft of the penis backward by incising the skin and reapproximating it. This is called *peno-scrotal webbing*. It is not uncommon, though the increase in apparent length is often minimal and certainly not enough to recommend this procedure on a regular basis.

Surgical Procedures for Girth

To increase the girth of the penis, physicians have injected silicone around the base of the penis to give the appearance of larger girth and, by doing so, increase the friction during intercourse. More recently, some surgeons have actually aspirated fat from the buttocks and other fatty areas of the body by liposuction and injected this under the skin of the penis to give the appearance of a fatter, thicker penis. The problem with this technique is that the fat gets reabsorbed and may even become infected, resulting in a nodular penis. This can actually alter the shape and appearance of the penis. The complication increases as the amount of fat used increases.

Another technique to increase penile girth is a dermal fat graft. This technique utilizes taking a piece of skin with the underlying fat from the buttocks. The skin is cut off, and the thickened piece of remaining fat is wrapped under the skin of the penis to increase its girth. Again this is a major surgical procedure and should be done only by very experienced surgeons. These procedures are controversial and should really be reserved for a limited group of patients and done by urologists experienced in this technique. My feeling is that these procedures have no role in modern therapy for erectile dysfunction.

Some men will always be dissatisfied with the length

J.F. presented the office in severe distress. When he was having intercourse with his wife, he felt that she was looking at him in a different way. Apparently she had been with another man, and he felt she was dissatisfied with him because of the length of his penis. He spent a fair amount of time discussing the length of his penis, how it was inadequate for her pleasure, and how he had always been embarrassed in the locker room or the shower. Upon examination, he was a very robust man whose penis actually appeared larger than most men's penises, both in length and girth. He stated that his erect penis measured somewhere around 8 inches. My recommendation was not to have surgery, and I gave him the appropriate literature surrounding this, but he was quite unhappy. Unfortunately, he went elsewhere for an enlarging procedure.

of their penis, just as some women are unhappy about their breast size. I consider this to be strictly a cosmetic issue. I do not believe that a penile-lengthening procedure is indicated today. As physicians, our job is to counsel patients to prevent them from ending up with a disastrous complication and something less than what they started with. The cost of enlarging procedures has been variable, but it may cost up to $15,000 and it is done on an outpatient basis. If a patient wished to consider this operation, in addition to my recommending against it, I would probably recommend counseling in this regard.

Take-Home Points

- The best way to increase your penile length is to lose weight.

- The current operations that exist for lengthening the penis do not provide dramatic increase in length.

Chapter 10
New Treatments

T he next several years will completely change the way we approach both the diagnosis and treatment of sexual dysfunction for both men and women. New medications that will soon be available will change this field forever. As we learn more about the problem we learn more about prevention of the problem. While not increasing the length of life, these new treatments will dramatically improve the quality of life.

Medications

One new feature of erectile dysfunction treatment is medications. The following is by no means an exhaustive list, and numerous other medications are still on the horizon. Within ten years, literally dozens of these types of drugs will be available to choose from, not only for the primary treatment, but for the prevention of erectile dysfunction in younger men and in men who are at risk for erectile dysfunction.

During the normal erection, the release of nitric oxide stimulates the production of cyclic GMP. By increasing the amount of cyclic GMP, this causes the smooth muscle cells of the penis to relax and produce an erection. There are two ways to stimulate this. One way is to prevent the breakdown of cyclic GMP, and the other way is to cause more cyclic GMP to be made.

Viagra™

The approval of sildenafil (Viagra™) by the Food and Drug Administration ushers in a new era in the treatment of erectile dysfunction. Viagra™ is an enzyme blocker that causes increased levels of cyclic GMP. This is a tremendously complicated way to say that this drug prevents the breakdown of a metabolite that causes an erection. Viagra™ is the first truly effective oral agent for male erectile dysfunction.

For most patients, the recommended dosage is 50 mg, taken orally approximately one hour before sexual activity. It may be taken as early as thirty minutes or as long as four hours before anticipated sexual activity, but the drug has no effect without sexual stimulation. The medication comes in three strengths, 25-, 50-, and 100-mg tablets.

When Viagra™ is administered properly, it proves to be remarkably effective. Significantly, it retains a half-life (the length of time the drug remains in the body) of up to four hours—long enough to allow for the additional, oft-noted side effect of more pronounced morning erections. Extensive studies on the drug conclude that it is broken down in the liver. The majority of the medication is then excreted from the body into the feces.

The major contraindications to this medication include men taking oral nitrates for the treatment of heart disease. The concern here is potential low blood pressure. Side effects are not severe or common but may include headaches, flushing, upset stomach, and nasal congestion. At higher doses, there may be some complaint about vision. No cases of priapism were reported during the clinical trials.

After a thorough history and physical examination, Viagra™ should be the first starting point in treating men with erectile dysfunction. Although it will not be effective for all men, clinical studies indicate that in a group of men with varying degrees of erectile dysfunction, up to 82 percent achieve good clinical response.

Interestingly, there are reports that this medication can be also effective for female patients with sexual dysfunction. This is, of course, an off-label use and requires careful counseling about the potential risks and benefits to the patient. The approval of this medication will begin a long line of oral agents that will dramatically change the way erectile dysfunction is diagnosed and treated, and it will shift the focus from treatment to prevention.

Phentolamine

Another new medication that will soon be available orally is phentolamine. This drug blocks the nervous system which, as a secondary response, relaxes the cavernosal smooth muscle wall. Phentolamine has also proven to be safe and effective, and it is currently undergoing testing in the United States.

This is not a new drug, and it has been marketed for many decades for high blood pressure and for use in rare tumors that produce high levels of stress hormones causing high blood pressure. Currently, phentolamine is a fast-release tablet formulation which reaches rapid blood levels. Major side effects include rapid heart rate and some expected nasal stuffiness. Phentolamine will soon be part of the armamentarium in the treatment of men with mild to moderate erectile dysfunction.

Apomorphine

Another new medication that will soon be available is apomorphine, a by-product of morphine, which is used to block dopamine receptors in the central nervous system. This particular compound is administered by placing it under the tongue, and it is also under testing. The results indicate good effectiveness in men with mild to moderate erectile dysfunction. The only major side effects of apomorphine therapy are yawning and nausea and, occasionally, vomiting.

Forskolin

Another medication, although not new, but currently available, is the drug Forskolin. This is an extract from the root of the herb coleus, a plant that has been used medically for generations. Apparently, Forskolin increases the levels of cyclic cAMP, which also helps to improve the quality of a drug-induced erection. This is currently available, but it is important that physicians inform their patients that Forskolin is a plant-derivative and has not been FDA approved for use in humans.

E.F. was a thirty-one-year-old man who had an unusually long and thin penis. While he was quite thin, his female partner weighed well over 200 pounds. While having intercourse with her assuming the superior position, his penis became dislodged, and she thought she had reinserted into the vaginal opening but had missed and snapped the penis in half. It tore both corporal bodies as well as the urethral body almost in two. There was a loud snap, extreme pain, and the penis became acutely angulated and black and blue. This required an urgent surgical procedure.

Prevention

Prevention is the best form of therapy. It is extremely important that young men are educated properly to allow them to develop habits that foster a preventive attitude.

The smooth muscle cells in the penis are finicky. They require "exercise," plenty of oxygen, low fat, and a healthy lifestyle. When the penis is not erect, it does not get a great deal of blood flow and, consequently, not a great deal of oxygen. When there is no oxygen, the smooth muscle cells are not nourished and, therefore, become replaced with scar tissue. The way to encourage penile oxygenation is by achieving erections—there is no other way. The penis equivalent of yawning is a nighttime erection. There are two ways to get erections: one is by having frequent sex or masturbating; the second is to get plenty of sleep so that you can have those nighttime erections that nourish the penis with oxygen.

Avoid bicycles. Irwin Goldstein, M.D., has been speaking out against bicycle seats. He has done extensive studies and has found that the typical narrow unpadded bicycle seats so common today support only 11 percent of a man's body weight and can totally cut off blood supply to the cavernosal arteries. I have seen several young men as patients who ride horses or do other types of straddling activity on a regular basis, and who, as a consequence, achieve poor erections. A good rule of thumb is to avoid sitting or straddling something where all the weight is between your legs and could potentially compress the penile artery.

Another very important lesson is to be gentle with your penis during sexual intercourse. When a penis is erect, even though it is hard, it is still a sensitive, blood-filled dynamic structure that is quite vulnerable to injury. It is not designed to have a partner on top, gyrating in numerous positions. Although "textbooks" commonly show various positions, it is important to avoid torque forces on the penis. I have seen several cases of penile fracture due to this. In this situation, the penis is erect and the partner is almost always on top. The penis becomes dislodged during intercourse and, in an attempt to reinsert it, the female partner will come down with all her weight. If she fails to insert the penis into her vaginal opening, she will acutely bend it against her pelvic bone. There will be a loud snap and extreme pain. This constitutes a surgical emergency and, if not dealt with immediately, can result in the permanent loss of erections.

Finally, medications will soon be available for prophylaxis. These medications will increase the levels of compounds that will improve the blood supply to the penis and will forestall or even prevent damage to the corporal smooth muscle that limits the ability to achieve an erection. This is essentially a reversal of the aging process. The future of erections is indeed exciting.

Female Sexual Dysfunction

Part of the ongoing revolution in sexual dysfunction is the realization that women, too, have sexual dysfunction. For many years this was always associated with many jokes and comments. Postmenopausal women frequently complain of vaginal dryness, difficulty of penetration, and decreased sexual interest and drive. This was always felt to have a hormonal basis and was subsequently treated hormonally. It is interesting to note that the use of the female hormone replacement is currently one of the best-selling drugs in the United States.

As the groundswell encouraging research and study into female sexual dysfunction gathers strength, then, will women come to reap the benefits of fuller, more satisfying sex lives? Medical researchers believe that will indeed be the case. In fact, in the near future, hundreds of thousands of women may come to learn what their partners already know: That Viagra™ can be of great help to their sexual problems. Some physicians have already started prescribing it on an "off-label" basis (in other words, for a use not specified by the manufacturer) to a number of women.

Admittedly, though, the jury is still out on that issue. This much, however, is fact: A Boston University study is currently underway to determine whether or not Viagra™ can help restore the sexual pleasure among those women who are taking it. And Viagra's™ manufacturer, Pfizer, Inc., is now in the midst of clinical trials among 500 women in the United Kingdom. If the studies prove successful—and many believe that they show every promise of doing so—the tests will soon be expanded to include thousands of women under the tough protocols required for FDA approval.

Many of the problems that affect men affect women on an equal basis. Female sexual dysfunction is associated with increased age, menopause, hysterectomy, and other vascular risk factors that include smoking, high blood pressure and its treatment, diabetes, and poor lifestyle habits: high-fat diet and overall lack of exercise.

Until now, nobody has focused on female sexual dysfunction as an actual problem. The real difficulty lies in the evaluation of the end response. In men this is easy. A firm erection and ejaculation provides an obvious way to monitor the effectiveness of drugs and treatments. Unlike the penis, the vagina does not have a tough outer membrane to trap blood. However, many of the same muscles that are present in men are present in women as well. The vagina, much like the male sexual organs, has tremendous innervation. The clitoris is the erectile body in women. It can become firm from increased blood flow and plays a role in orgasm as well. The primary function of the increased blood flow in the vagina is to provide fluid. Failure of this was erroneously thought to be the result of glands in the vagina, but in actuality, fluid fails to leak across and create the fluid necessary for vaginal lubrication and painless penile penetration.

Many of the new drugs currently available will have tremendous use for women as well as men. This, based on our understanding of the physiology and future research, will forever change our view of female sexual dysfunction.

Glossary

Aldomet: a medication used to treat high blood pressure that can cause erectile dysfunction.

Alpha receptor: the area where brain chemicals stimulate the nerve.

AMS: American Medical Systems, the company that makes penile prostheses.

Androgens: the overall classification of steroids that includes the hormone testosterone.

Apomorphine: a new medication to help men achieve an erection. This medication is currently under intensive studies.

Arteriography: a technique where a catheter is inserted into the artery and contrast material is inserted to visualize an arterial blockage.

Cavernosal artery: this is the artery that is the main blood supply to the corporal body of the penis. It is readily visualized during a Doppler examination. This artery will dilate when the blood flow increases.

Cavernosography: a technique where contrast material is inserted into the cavernosal body and an X ray is taken in order to identify a venous leak. This is generally done just prior to corrective surgery.

Cavernosometry: a technique where a saline solution is inserted into the cavernosal body at a given rate to measure the pressure in order to determine the magnitude of the venous leak.

Corpora cavernosa: the anatomic part of the penis that contains the smooth muscle fibers. The outer lining of the structure is very tough.

Doppler duplex examination: an ultrasound examination using a special probe to visualize the amount of blood flow to the penis. It is currently the best available technique for the diagnostic workup of erectile dysfunction.

Duraphase: the semi rigid prosthesis that is movable.

Emission: the deposition of semen into the posterior urethra prior to ejaculation.

Finasteride: a commonly used medication to shrink the prostate. It is in the class of five alpha-reductase inhibitors.

Hyperprolactinemia: the state of elevated prolactin in the body, frequently associated with decreased libido.

Hypospadias: a congenital abnormality in which the urinary opening on the penis is moved to the undersurface.

Papaverine: a derivative of the poppy seed. It is nonnarcotic. It is used to inject into the penis to produce an erection.

Peyronie's disease: a condition that causes scarring in the wall of the corporal body. It is associated with bending, pain, and erectile dysfunction.

Phentolamine: an alpha blocker previously used for the treatment of blood pressure and more recently has been used to inject into the penis. A newer formulation is currently under intensive study by the FDA for use as an oral medication.

Priapism: a painful erection that lasts for more than four hours and is not associated with sexual desire.

Prostaglandin: a medication injected into the penis to produce an erection.

Prosthesis: a device that is surgically inserted into the penis to produce an erection.

Psychogenic erectile dysfunction: the primary cause erectile dysfunction not related to a definable organic medical problem.

Rigiscan: a device used to perform nocturnal penile tumescence monitoring.

Testosterone: the hormone involved both with sexual function and fertility.

Trazodone: a drug used to treat depression and occasionally used to treat erectile dysfunction; its major side effect is priapism.

Tumescence: blood flow to the penis that causes an increase in diameter and length but is not associated with rigidity.

Tunica albuginea: a tough outer covering of the corporal body.

Vacuum erection device (VED): a device used to create an erection without the use of medications or surgery.

Yohimbine: a medication used to treat erections. It is an herb that has been used for centuries.

Appendix A

International Index of Erectile Function (IIEF) Questionnaire

Investigator _____ Date of Visit ___/___/___
                                        (month/day/year)

Please use a cross mark ⊗ where applicable and be sure to initial and date all corrections

○ Not Done   Subject Questionnaire - Section 1

Instructions: These questions ask about the effects your erection problems have had on your sex life, *over the past 4 weeks.* Please answer the following questions as honestly and clearly as possible. In answering these questions the following definitions apply:

 Sexual activity includes intercourse, caressing, foreplay, and masturbation

 Sexual intercourse is defined as vaginal penetration of the partner (you entered your partner)

 Sexual stimulation includes situations like foreplay with a partner, looking at erotic pictures, etc.

 Ejaculate is defined as the ejection of semen from the penis (or the feeling of this)

Source: *The International Index of Erectile Function (IIEF): A Multidimensional Scale for Assessment of Erectile Dysfunction.* By Raymond C. Rosen, Alan Riley, Gorm Wagner, Ian H. Osterloh, John Kirkpatrick, and Avanish Mishra. Copyright 1997 by Elsevier Science, Inc.

Check ONLY one box per question:

1. *Over the past 4 weeks*, how often were you able to get an erection during sexual activity?

○ No sexual activity
○ Almost always or always
○ Most times (much more than half the time)
○ Sometimes (about half the time)
○ A few times (much less than half the time)
○ Almost never or never

2. *Over the past 4 weeks*, when you had erections with sexual stimulation, how often were your erections hard enough for penetration?

○ No sexual stimulation
○ Almost always or always
○ Most times (much more than half the time)
○ Sometimes (about half the time)
○ A few times (much less than half the time)
○ Almost never or never

Questions 3, 4, and 5 will ask about erections you may have had during sexual intercourse.

3. *Over the past 4 weeks*, when you attempted sexual intercourse, how often were you able to penetrate (enter) your partner?

○ Did not attempt intercourse
○ Almost always or always
○ Most times (much more than half the time)
○ Sometimes (about half the time)
○ A few times (much less than half the time)
○ Almost never or never

4. *Over the past 4 weeks*, during sexual intercourse, <u>how often</u> were you able to maintain your erection after you had penetrated (entered) your partner?

○ Did not attempt intercourse
○ Almost always or always
○ Most times (much more than half the time)
○ Sometimes (about half the time)
○ A few times (much less than half the time)
○ Almost never or never

5. *Over the past 4 weeks*, during sexual intercourse, <u>how difficult</u> was it to maintain your erection to completion of intercourse?

○ Did not attempt intercourse
○ Extremely difficult
○ Very difficult
○ Difficult
○ Slightly difficult
○ Not difficult

6. *Over the past 4 weeks*, how many times have you attempted sexual intercourse?

○ No attempts
○ 1–2 attempts
○ 3–4 attempts
○ 5–6 attempts
○ 7–10 attempts
○ 11 or more attempts

7. *Over the past 4 weeks*, when you attempted sexual intercourse how often was it satisfactory for <u>you</u>?

○ Did not attempt intercourse
○ Almost always or always
○ Most times (much more than half the time)
○ Sometimes (about half the time)
○ A few times (much less than half the time)
○ Almost never or never

8. *Over the past 4 weeks*, how much have you enjoyed sexual intercourse?

○ No intercourse
○ Very highly enjoyable
○ Highly enjoyable
○ Fairly enjoyable
○ Not very enjoyable
○ Not enjoyable

9. *Over the past 4 weeks*, when you had sexual stimulation <u>or</u> intercourse how often did you ejaculate?

○ Did not attempt intercourse
○ Almost always or always
○ Most times (much more than half the time)
○ Sometimes (about half the time)
○ A few times (much less than half the time)
○ Almost never or never

10. *Over the past 4 weeks*, when you had sexual stimulation <u>or</u> intercourse how often did you have the feeling of orgasm or climax (with or without ejaculation)?

○ No sexual stimulation or intercourse
○ Almost always or always
○ Most times (much more than half the time)
○ Sometimes (about half the time)
○ A few times (much less than half the time)
○ Almost never or never

Questions 11 and 12 ask about sexual desire.

Let's define *sexual desire* as a feeling that may include wanting to have a sexual experience (for example, masturbation or intercourse), thinking about having sex, or feeling frustrated due to a lack of sex.

11. *Over the past 4 weeks*, how often have you felt <u>sexual desire</u>?

○ Almost always or always
○ Most times (much more than half the time)
○ Sometimes (about half the time)
○ A few times (much less than half the time)
○ Almost never or never

12. *Over the past 4 weeks*, how would you rate your level of <u>sexual desire</u>?

○ Very high
○ High
○ Moderate
○ Low
○ Very low or none at all

13. *Over the past 4 weeks*, how satisfied have you been with your overall <u>sex life</u>?

○ Very satisfied
○ Moderately satisfied
○ About equally satisfied and dissatisfied
○ Moderately dissatisfied
○ Very dissatisfied

14. *Over the past 4 weeks*, how satisfied have you been with your <u>sexual relationship</u> with your partner?

○ Very satisfied
○ Moderately satisfied
○ About equally satisfied and dissatisfied
○ Moderately dissatisfied
○ Very dissatisfied

15. *Over the past 4 weeks*, how do you rate your <u>confidence</u> that you can get and keep your erection?

○ Very high
○ High
○ Moderate
○ Low
○ Very low

Sexual activity includes intercourse, caressing, foreplay, and masturbation

Sexual intercourse is defined as vaginal penetration of the partner (you entered your partner)

Sexual stimulation includes situations like foreplay with a partner, looking at erotic pictures, etc.

Ejaculate is defined as the ejection of semen from the penis (or the feeling of this)

Scoring Algorithm for IIEF

All items are scored in 5 domains as follows:

Domain	Items	Score Range	Max Score
Erectile Function	1,2,3, 4,5,15	0–5	30
Orgasmic Function	9,10	0–5	10
Sexual Desire	11,12	1–5	10
Intercourse Satisfaction	6,7,8	0–5	15
Overall Satisfaction	13,14	1–5	10

Clinical Interpretation:

I. Erectile function total scores can be interpreted as follows:

Score	Interpretation
0–6	Severe dysfunction
7–12	Moderate dysfunction
13–18	Mild-to-moderate dysfunction
19–24	Mild dysfunction
25–30	No dysfunction

II. Orgasmic function total scores can be interpreted as follows:

Score	Interpretation
0–2	Severe dysfunction
3–4	Moderate dysfunction
5–6	Mild-to-moderate dysfunction
7–8	Mild dysfunction
9–10	No dysfunction

III. <u>Sexual desire</u> total scores can be interpreted as follows:

Score	Interpretation
0–2	Severe dysfunction
3–4	Moderate dysfunction
5–6	Mild-to-moderate dysfunction
7–8	Mild dysfunction
9–10	No dysfunction

IV. <u>Intercourse satisfaction</u> total scores can be interpreted as follows:

Score	Interpretation
0–3	Severe dysfunction
4–6	Moderate dysfunction
7–9	Mild-to-moderate dysfunction
10–12	Mild dysfunction
13–15	No dysfunction

V. <u>Overall satisfaction</u> total scores can be interpreted as follows:

Score	Interpretation
0–2	Severe dysfunction
3–4	Moderate dysfunction
5–6	Mild-to-moderate dysfunction
7–8	Mild dysfunction
9–10	No dysfunction

Appendix B

NIH Consensus Statement on Impotence

Impotence, which affects about 30 million men in the United States, is the consistent inability to attain and maintain a penile erection sufficient to permit satisfactory sexual intercourse. An erection results from a complex interaction between muscles, nerves, and blood vessels and is influenced by psychological and behavioral factors.

Men who see impotence as a natural consequence of aging may change their sexual expectations and behavior. Increasingly, however, men are seeking treatments to restore erectile function, while the medical community has not generally agreed on when to perform certain tests and offer specific treatments. Therefore, the National Institute of Diabetes and Digestive and Kidney Diseases and the NIH Office of Medical Applications of Research held a Consensus Development Conference on Impotence, December 7–9, 1992.

The panel of specialists in urology, nursing, endocrinology, cardiology, gerontology, psychology, psychiatry, epidemiology, biostatistics, and a representative of the general public arrived at the following conclusions.

Because the term impotence has significant negative overtones and has been used to describe a range of sexual problems, the panel favored using the specific term "erectile dysfunction."

The risk of erectile dysfunction increases with age, but men who have diabetes, hypertension, high cholesterol, low high-density lipoproteins, Peyronie's disease, priapism, depression, injuries or disorders affecting the nerves or blood vessels, or who take prescription or other drugs are also at risk. Though cigarette smoking does not directly cause erectile dysfunction, it can increase the risk of vascular disease and hypertension.

Because erectile dysfunction is most often the result of a combination of psychological and physical factors, education about anxiety's role may help prevent or reduce the duration and severity of erectile dysfunction.

For men complaining of erectile dysfunction, the panel recommended a careful, detailed medical and sexual history, followed by a physical examination and basic laboratory studies to identify psychological factors as well as unrecognized disease.

The panel emphasized that a sexual history, an often neglected element of the evaluation, is vital to assess a man's true complaint, expectations, and motivation for further diagnosis and treatment. The sexual partner's perceptions should also be obtained if possible.

The physical examination should include the testicles, penis, prostate, anal sphincter tone, femoral and lower extremity pulses, and neurologic examination of perianal sensation and bulbocavernosus reflex. Suspected neurological problems may require more extensive tests.

Laboratory studies should include a urinalysis and blood tests for complete blood count, creatinine, lipid profile, fasting blood sugar, thyroid function, and morning testosterone. Low testosterone indicates a second test for this hormone, and luteinizing hormone and prolactin should also be measured.

The panel identified additional tests that might be useful in some men.

Nocturnal penile tumescence testing may be useful in

men who report a complete absence of erections or when a primarily psychogenic cause is suspected.

Only men who are seriously considering penile injections, implants, or vascular surgery require intracavernous pharmacologic injection of a vasodilating agent to assess penile blood supply. If this test produces an erection, home penile injection therapy may be an option. However, anxiety or discomfort during the test may prevent an erection even in men who have adequate blood vessel function.

Duplex color ultrasonography, dynamic infusion pharmacocavernosometry and cavernosography, and pharmacologic pelvic/penile angiography will further define vascular disorders in young men who do not respond to the penile injection test, do have a history of perineal or pelvic trauma, and are serious candidates for vascular surgery. These tests are best done by experts in the vascular aspects of erectile dysfunction.

While the most common treatments—vacuum devices, injections, and implants—are effective in producing erections in most men, many discontinue their use. Treatment may be more successful when the sexual partner participates in evaluation and when treatment, beginning with the least risky, is tailored to the couple's goals. Counseling is always recommended.

Hormone-related erectile dysfunction is relatively rare, but in cases of confirmed low serum testosterone, the panel recommended intramuscular injections of testosterone enanthate or cypionate. In cases of confirmed hyperprolactinemia, the oral drug bromocryptine is appropriate. However, these treatments are inappropriate and may increase the risk of prostate cancer when testicular function is normal.

The panel found that while vacuum devices require manual dexterity, they are very effective in producing an erection and are relatively risk-free, although they may cause some discomfort and impair ejaculation.

The most effective agents for penile injection are papaverine, phentolamine, and prostaglandin E_1. They can be used in combination to reduce pain, penile corporal fibrosis, fibrotic nodules, and priapism. Injections can be a problem for men who have poor vision, poor manual dexterity, psychiatric disease, and for those who receive anticoagulant therapy or who cannot tolerate transient hypotension. In addition, drugs used to reverse priapism can cause death in men taking monoamine oxidase inhibitors for hypertension.

Mechanical failure, prosthesis-associated infection (most common in men with diabetes, spinal cord injuries, or urinary tract infections) and erosion can occur with rigid, malleable, or inflatable penile prosthetics. Inflatable implants produce the most natural flaccid and erect states, but also have the highest failure and reoperation rates. No problems related to silicone migration from these implants have been reported.

The panel recommended that vascular surgery, which is often unsuccessful, be done only in a clinical research setting on young men who have congenital vascular defects or who have had pelvic or penile injuries.

Because of widespread ignorance, misinformation, and embarrassment about erectile dysfunction, the panel encouraged dissemination of information through the media, community, and health organizations, and called for required education in human sexuality for health professionals.

Finally, the panel encouraged a multi-disciplinary approach to future investigations and urged researchers to develop diagnostic and treatment outcome standards. They also recommended epidemiological studies; studies on the racial, cultural, ethnic, and social perceptions and expectations of erectile function and dysfunction; studies to identify means to prevent erectile dysfunction; and clinical trials to assess and compare behavioral, mechanical, pharmacologic, and surgical treatments.

This conference was cosponsored by the National Institute of Neurological Disorders and Stroke and the National Institute on Aging.

NIH Consensus Development Conference
December 7–9, 1992
Office of Medical Applications of Research
National Institutes of Health

Free, single copies of the complete NIH Consensus Statement on Impotence may be ordered from the Office of Medical Applications of Research, National Institutes of Health, Federal Building, Room 618, Bethesda, Maryland 20892, phone (301) 496-1143.

Index